IT'S ALL ABOUT CHOICE™

Getting Back in the Game!

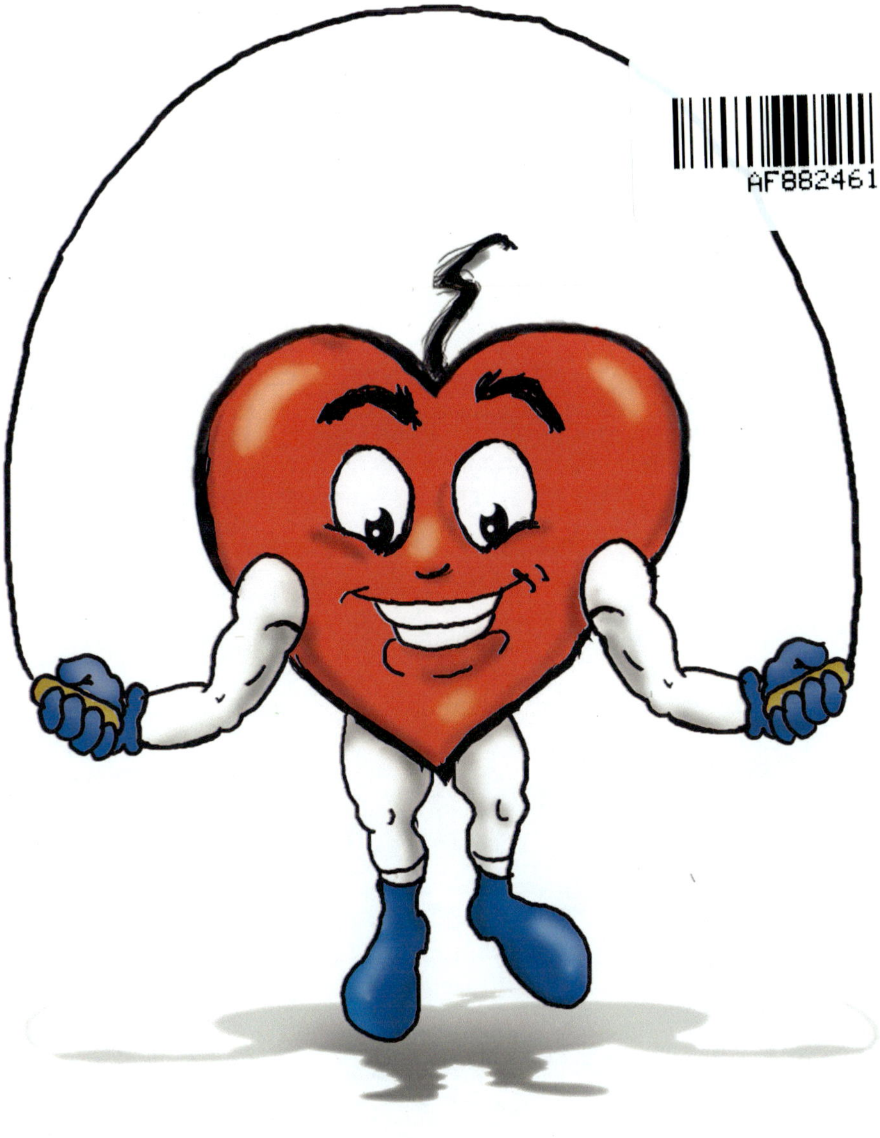

Featuring the Cardio Kidd

by Herb D. Trainer

AF882461

DEDICATION

It's All About Choice: Getting Back in the Game! is dedicated to my mom, Faye Benjamin, who unfortunately departed this world January 2, 2010. She was my biggest fan and cheerleader, and constantly stayed on my case about completing this project. The fact that she won't be here to witness the finished product or, more importantly, the potentially positive impact we both felt it would have for improving the physical and mental health of children worldwide, is my one huge regret.

Her favorite part of the book—the "Healthy Choices" rap song—always made her smile. Her favorite character was Mr. Stuffin-Gutt. She was a big kid at heart, and most kids love good rhyming. She had a wicked, razor sharp sense of humor. When she got on a roll, she'd make you laugh hard all day. That's probably one of the things about her I miss the most.

Well Moms, if you're watching over my shoulder, I made good on my promise to you. I am sorry I didn't get it done sooner. But had it not been for your strong, relentless encouragement, *It's All About Choice* would have remained nothing but a dream.

–Love always!
Your son, Herb

Copyright © 2011 Herb D. Trainer
All rights reserved.

ISBN: 0615440797
ISBN-13: 9780615440798

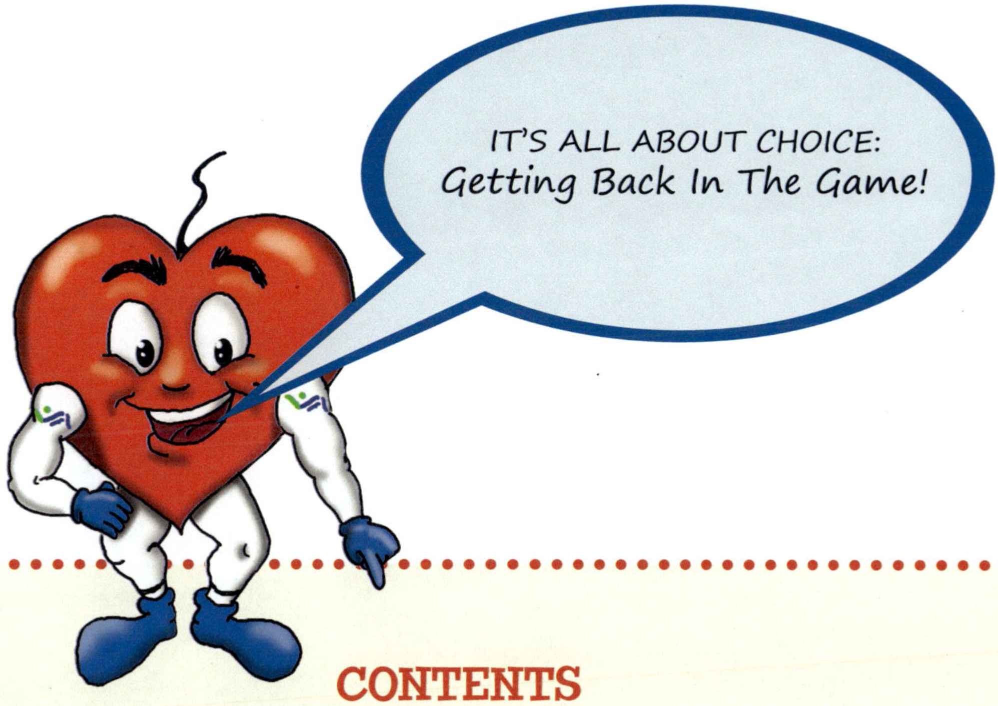

CONTENTS

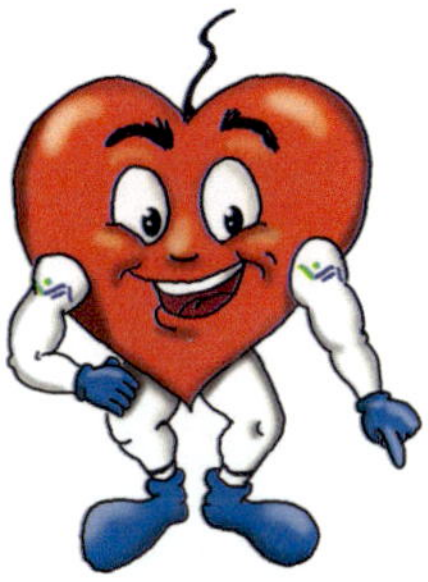

ACKNOWLEDGEMENTS

It would take a whole other book to thank all the friends and family who've played some part in helping me create *It's All About Choice: Getting Back in the Game*! So, forgive me if I fail to mention you if you're one of the contributors who helped me make this dream a reality.

Even though my mom is not here, at least physically, there's no question her inspiration and the confidence she expressed in my abilities kept me going, even when I was frustrated, tired, or couldn't think of the right words...Thanks, Momsy!

The following friends played a special role in the creation of the book you're about to read. I was very fortunate to find my gifted illustrator, Taillefer Long, aka TL. He not only created amazing and fun illustrations that brought all my colorful characters to life, he put his heart and soul in this project. I can't thank you enough.

Even though this is my first book, I thought I'd hit a home run. But I wasn't sure, so I asked Susie Wilde, a superb writer's coach, for her thoughts. Well, it turns out I had hit something closer to a double—at best. It was humbling to get all those red marks on my "great" manuscript. Susie forced me to bring out more of every character's personality, and tie up several loose ends in the story. Thanks so much!

Producing the rap song that I wrote to make this project truly unique was a challenge in itself. The first producer disappeared in the middle of the production. Then I found the Apple Juice Kid. He carefully picked up the pieces and brought together great talent such as Carlitta Durand and King Mez. He mixed the backbeat, and voilà—we had a toe-tapping, head-bopping rap song with a positive message! Thanks Carlitta, King Mez, and AJ!

When I needed straight-up feedback on anything from cover design to the storyline, I couldn't ask for a sharper mind or more vocal cheerleader than my sage cousin, Yvonne Pugh, Esq. And my cousin, Dwight Manning, has been a steady rock of support!

The folks I train to help improve their health and fitness are also my friends. And they all were inspirational to me. Some, however, were exceptional in their support such as Doug Durrett, who found time in his busy schedule to bring me articles, provide

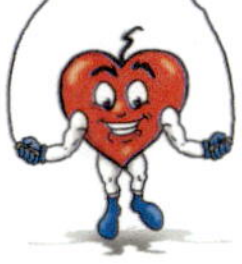

names of potential endorsers or sponsors. Another source of great inspiration and encouragement was Kathy Mills who sometimes showed more enthusiasm for my book and its healthy choices message than I did. Thank you my friends!

Of course, every man needs a partner by his side. For the past 11 years Barbara Hershey was there for me. No words will ever come close to expressing my gratitude for everything she's done to support my dream.

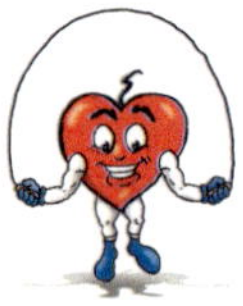

INTRODUCTION

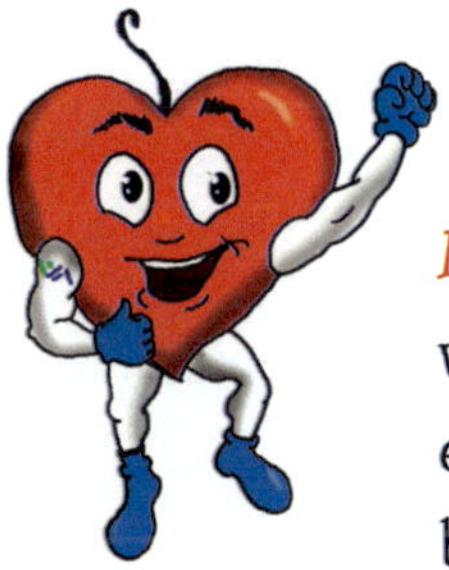

It's All About Choice (IAAC): Getting Back in the Game! is a children's book with colorful fictional characters that deliver both empowering and life-enhancing messages. The story centers on the struggles of an overweight boy who is humiliated and bullied by other kids when he returns to the basketball court—in a new neighborhood—after a year of avoiding the sport he loves. (You'll have to read the book to discover why he avoids the court.) And how, through hard work and discipline, he loses weight and gets back in the game. The book's health and fitness lessons and training are expressed in the form of two cool, positive rap songs and several rhymes. The Healthy Choices Rap is free to download at www.CardioKidd.com when you buy this book. You'll love the song's lyrics and catchy beat!

This children's book is intended to both increase awareness and promote healthy choice messages in a fun, colorful, and attention-grabbing way. The "bad" characters include a walking doughnut (Sweet Glazio), a chocolate chip cookie (Chubbalicious Chip), crinkle-cut, greasy french fry (Faz-n-Greazy), and an overstuffed stomach (Mr. Stuffin-Gutt), the leader of this trouble-making trio called the Blubba Hill Gang. The good guys are equally colorful.

Besides encouraging healthier food choices, regular exercise, and discouraging bullying, IAAC provides examples of forgiveness, conflict resolution and friendship between kids with different cultural backgrounds, to name but a few. I've also included discussion points for teachers/parents in appendix I. And all kids who read IAAC will have the chance to compete for great prizes in our first annual IAAC Essay and Rap Competition. Learn more about these programs at www.CardioKidd.com.

Getting Back in the Game has been strongly endorsed by teachers and parents. More importantly, I believe kids—worldwide—will love it! –Herb D Trainer

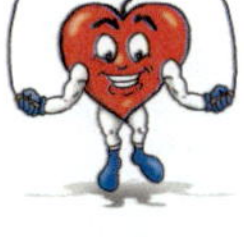

CHAPTER 1:
Getting Back in the Game!

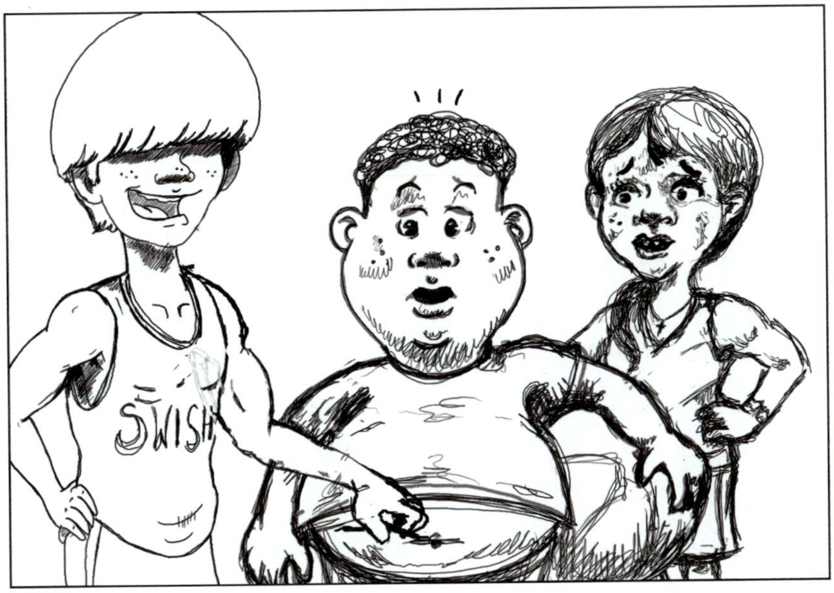

The Bully Setback

Danny thought a change of scenery would
help him get back in the game.
Only he wasn't prepared to get bullied
and wander the street in shame.

"Sheez, about time! I thought that bell would never ring," Danny Dixon fussed to himself, as he DASHED out of school and waddled home as fast as his pudgy legs would go.

"Danny! You're dripping with sweat. Why are you rush—"

"Hi Mom!" Danny, huffing and puffing, scooted past his mom, ran to his room, tossed his books on the bed, grabbed his basketball and ran past his mom again.

"Danny, here's some yummy snack choices. I baked your fav cookies, and there's pound cake left from yesterday."

"MMYOOOW!!!!" Danny's cat Dusty leaped straight up in the air.

"S-s-sorry Dusty! Bye Mom!"

"Danny wait! At least grab a cookie! How was your first day of school?"

"Great Mom! Please feed Dusty for me. See you later!"

Danny took off like he was chasing an ice cream truck. When he arrived at the park, Danny looked down and saw his heart pounding through his skin-tight, sweaty T-shirt. He leaned over and held his chest for several minutes until he caught his breath.

"This...is a...cool...park. Th...The courts are much...nicer...than my old park. Nice trees. Even new tennis courts. Oh man, it's been so long since I've been on a basketball court. It feels so good just to dribble the ball again."

Danny looked down at the court as if he wanted to kiss it and then up toward the sky, "I'm so sorry, Dad for not playing ball and gaining all this extra weight since you passed away last summer. I know I promised you that I'd keep working hard on the court and in the classroom, and take care of Mom. But it took a lot more time to get over the pain of losing you than I ever thought. Don't worry Dad, I'm ready to work my butt off like you taught me and make you proud."

Danny dribbled the ball between his legs and behind his back as he headed toward the courts when he spotted a rare sight.

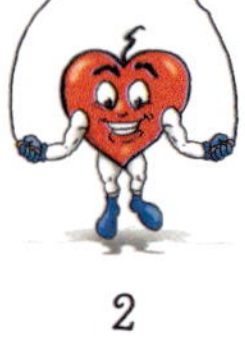

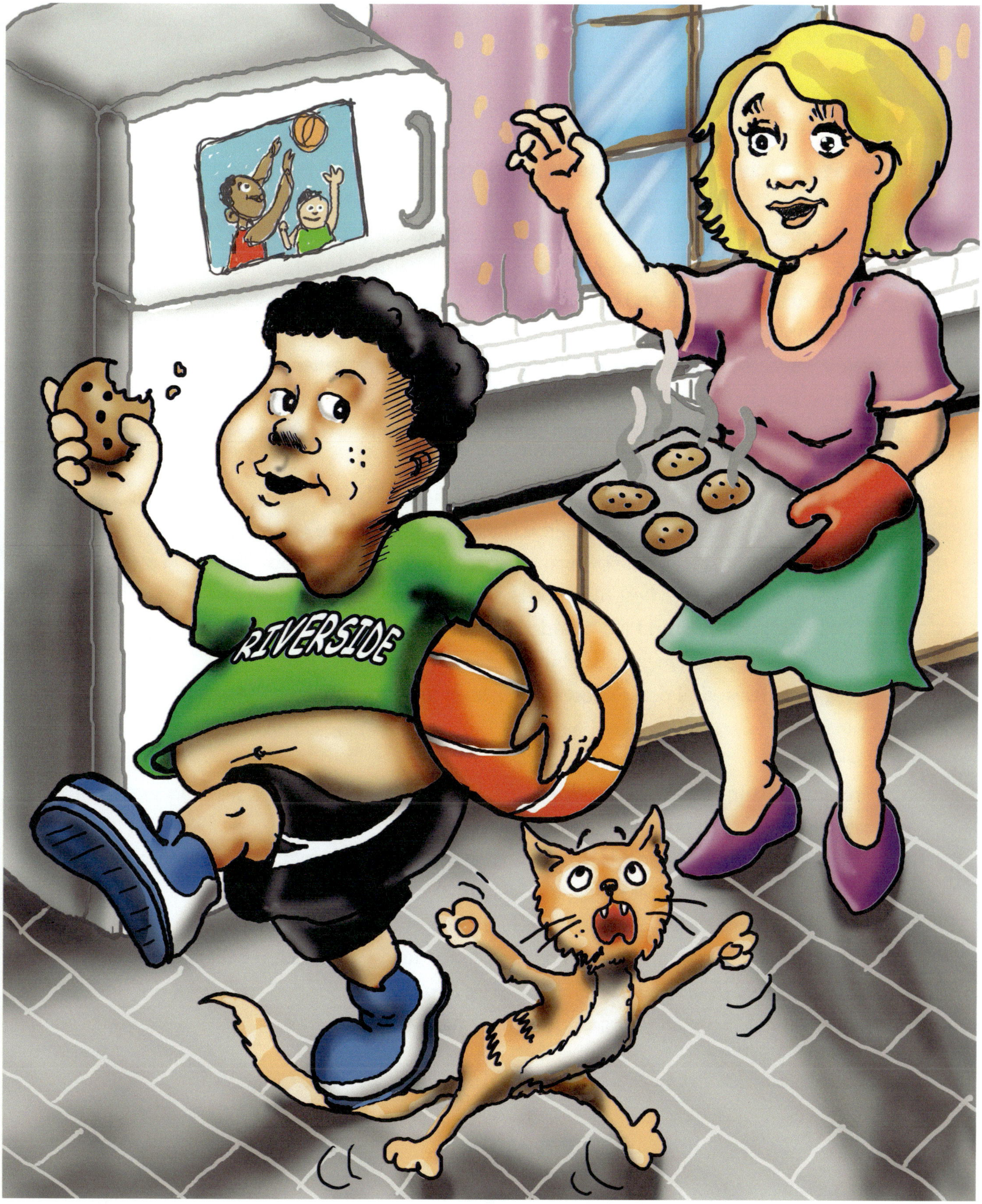
RIVERSIDE

"Wow! Wonder who that dark-haired cutie shooting alone on the other court is?" he said to himself. "Hmmm, I bet she's that star point guard that balls for Park City--her shooting and ball-handling skills are better than most guys!"

Danny, still dribbling, zigzagged his way toward Sonny McSwisher, one of the biggest boys shooting around on the court. "Hey, aren't you the captain of Park City's basketball team? Looks like you need another baller, can I play with your team?" Danny asked.

Swish turned his back on Danny and looked toward the girl who had caused Danny's eyes to twinkle.

"Hey Carmen!" Swish shouted. "We need one more baller to play!" Then Swish sneered at Danny, and pointed toward Carmen, "That's Carmen Acosta, Park City's best point guard and my next door neighbor since we played peek-a-boo together in diapers. If we need a baller, it'll be Carmen."

"But you already have ten Swish," Carmen shouted back. "I gotta practice for a big game against Mt. Baker—they crushed us in the championship game last year!"

Swish aimed his right index finger toward the basketball hoop, "C'mon lil sis, ONE game! We need the park's best ballhandler," Swish pleaded.

Carmen jogged over and half-nodded "Okay big bro, ONE game!"

Swish high-fived Carmen and whispered, "Hey, who's the doughboy?"

Carmen shrugged, "I don't know. Never seen him before."

Swish and Carmen walked over to Danny. "Hi, I'm Carmen, and this is my bestie Swish."

Instantly, Danny's mouth was dryer than day-old toast; his palms were so wet with sweat the basketball slipped out of his hands.

"My name is D-Dan, and uh...I just moved around the corner. If you need another baller, I was the top scorer at Riverside Academy."

Carmen glanced down at Danny's belly, which overlapped his shorts.

"Really? No offense Danny, but you look kinda heavy to be a top baller."

Danny sucked in his potbelly as much as he could, but it popped right back out when he spoke. "But...I...Look, if you just give me a chance."

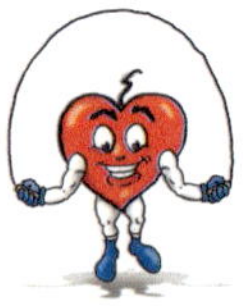

Then Swish reached out and grabbed a big chunk of Danny's flabby stomach, "C'mon, get real Chunky Dan, how you gonna run and jump with all these extra groceries jiggling like an over-filled water balloon? You sure you weren't looking for the SUMO wrestling team?"

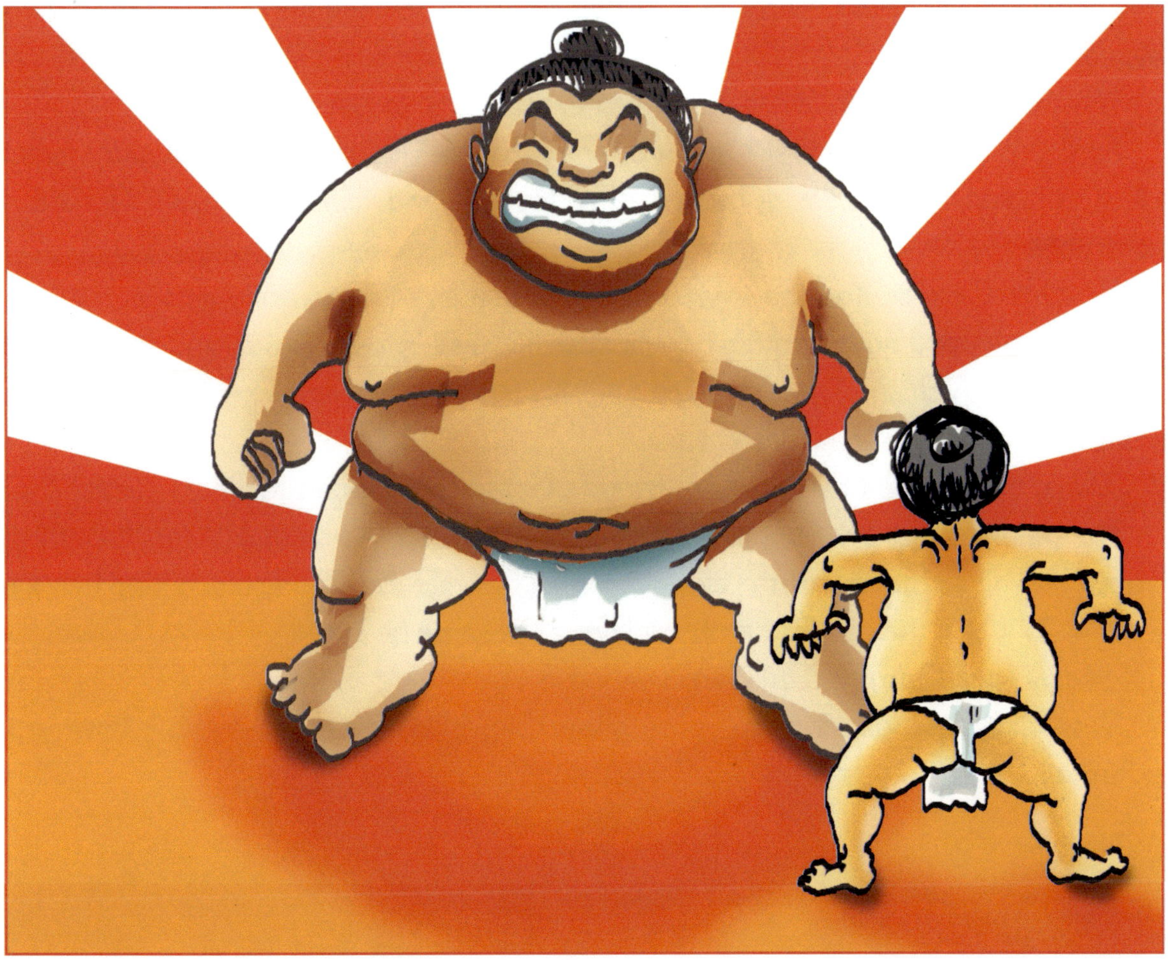

"Hey, don't pinch me, Swish!" Danny heard one laugh, then another, and by the time he looked up, all the players had joined in. Except Carmen. She must have seen the hurt look on Danny's pie-shaped face because she patted him on the back.

"Don't trip Danny," Carmen said. "Have a seat. You can take my spot next game."

"Thanks Carmen. I'm cool." But only a lip reader would have heard him. Like a leftover can of soda, Danny's bubbly spirit had lost all its fizzle. His head sank, and his shoulders drooped.

Carmen gave her old friend an icy glare and then scolded him like a puppy that just leaked on the carpet.

"That was very mean Swish. You need to apologize to Danny—now!"

As if she had spread a wet blanket over a campfire, the rip-roaring laughter faded to a few scattered crackles. Swish backed away, took a few dribbles, and made a long three-point shot.

"Ah chill, Carmen. You see any pampers on that boy? Everybody gets teased!"

Danny plopped down on the bench, sank his head into his hands, and stared blankly at the ground. A chain of ants crawled over his tennis shoes, carrying food crumbs, and working together like close teammates.

"Dang, even these tiny ants have friends. Not gonna happen for me, I guess."

The painful lump swelling in his throat made it hard to breath. His soft brown eyes looked like he had been cutting raw onions all day. He stood to leave, taking just a few seconds to watch the kids having fun playing the game he loved.

"See ya later, Chunky Dan!" Swish yelled.

"One day...One day I'm going to show Swish how wrong he is," Danny said to himself.

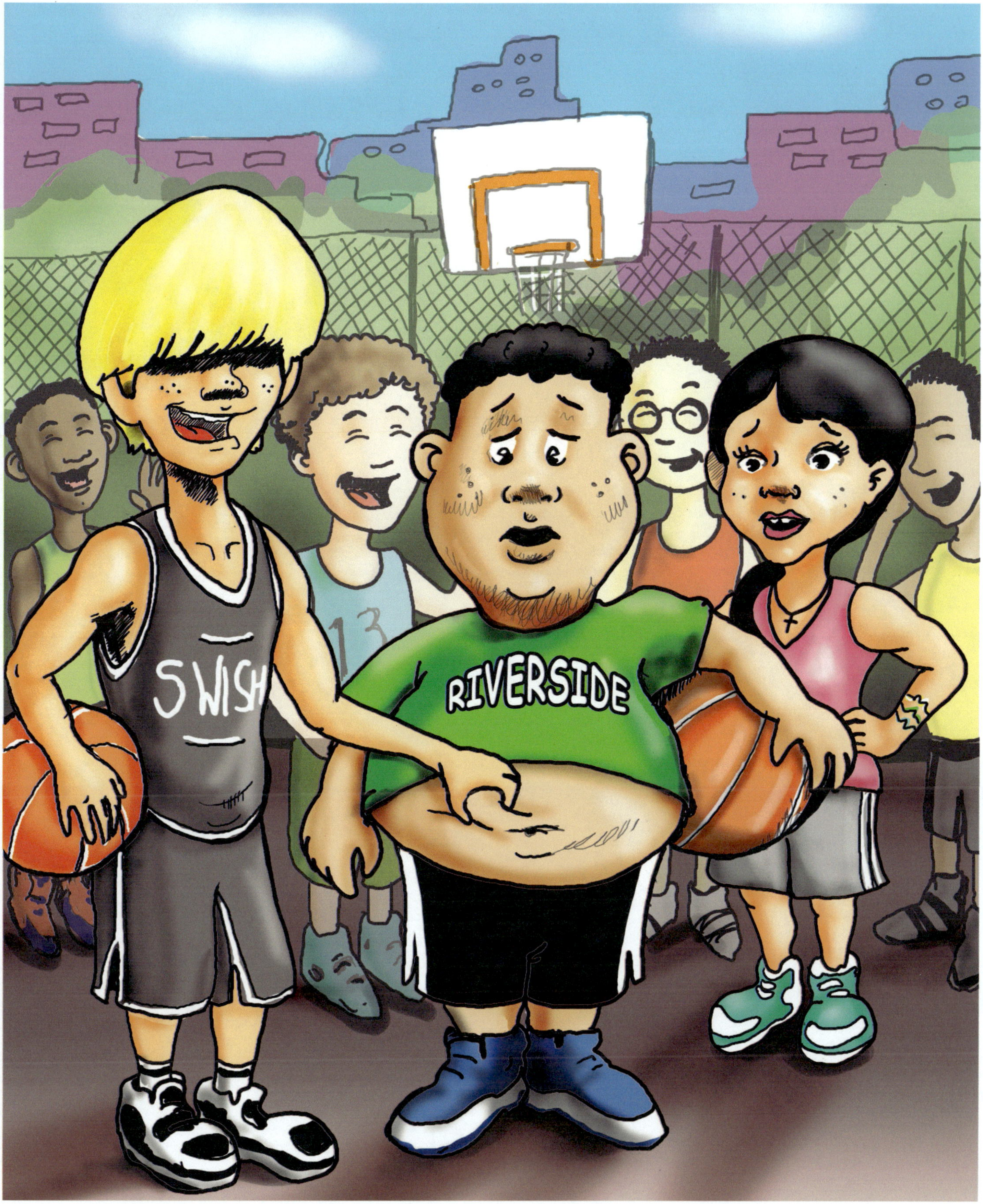
SWISH
13
RIVERSIDE

CHAPTER 2:
Getting Back in the Game!

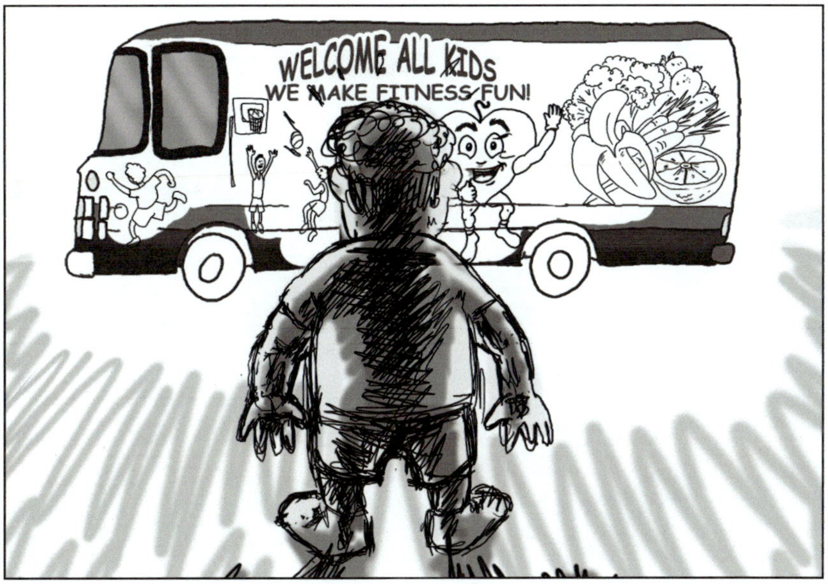

New Beginnings!

Danny wandered the street
feeling sad and very alone.
Those words "See-ya-later-Chunky-Dan"
cut like a knife,
all the way to the bone.

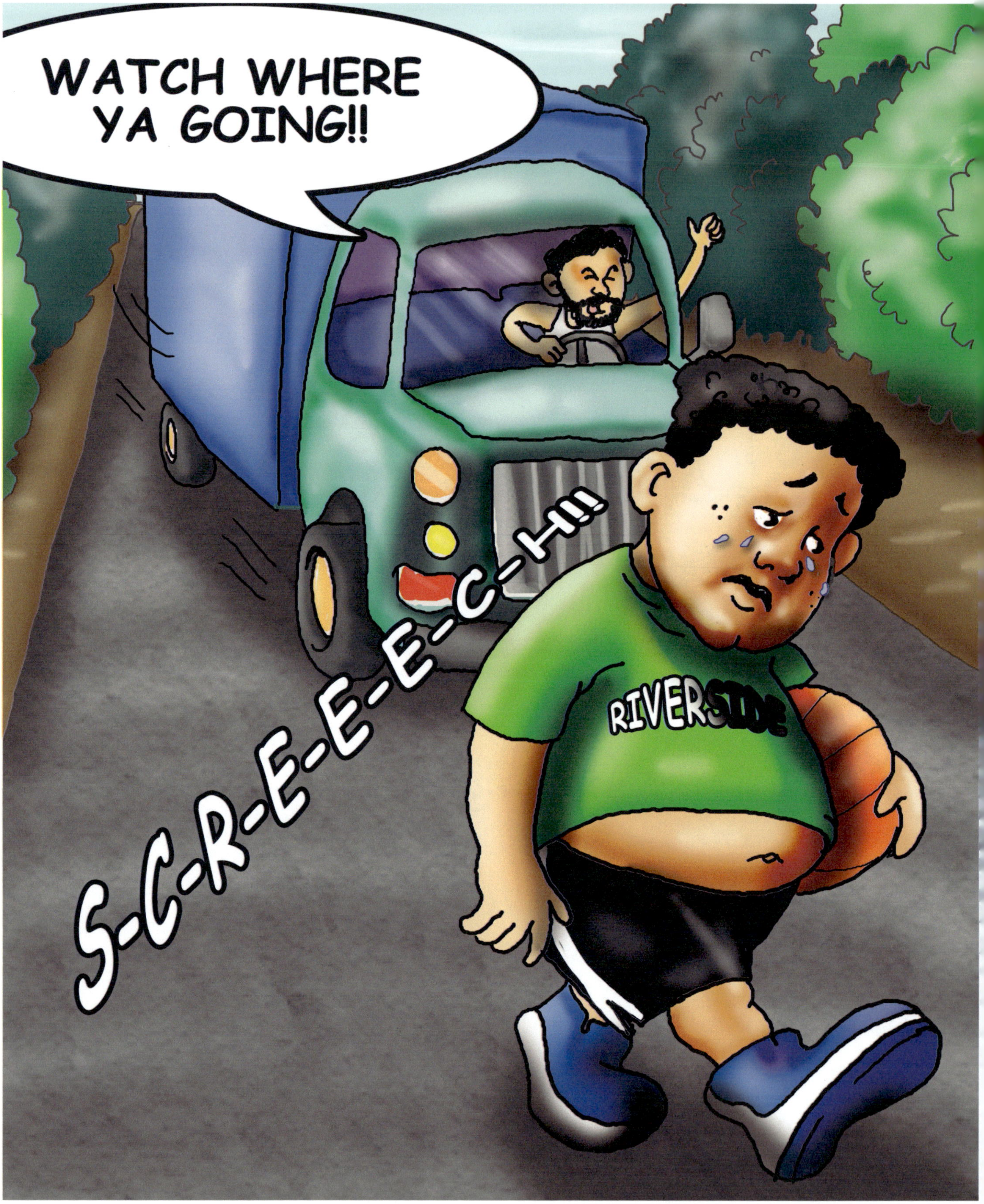
WATCH WHERE YA GOING!!
S-C-R-E-E-E-E-C-H!!
RIVERSIDE

As Danny passed a parked shiny black car, he caught a glimpse of his body's barrel-shaped reflection. He stopped. And stared. No amount of swallowing could hold back that hard painful lump in his throat. Tears streamed down his chubby cheeks faster than he could wipe them away.

"W-Why do I have to be so fat? WHY?"

S-c-r-e-e-e-c-h! Danny's head snapped up. His legs froze; beads of sweat burst out across his forehead, and his eyes bugged out. A huge truck was headed directly toward him; the driver managed to swerve at the last second, narrowly avoiding hitting him.

"Watch where ya going!" the driver yelled.

Danny tried to mumble an apology, but his tongue and body might as well have belonged to a storefront mannequin—until the moment he realized his new basketball was bouncing down the street.

"Noooooo!" Danny screamed. "Don't run over my..." Splaaat!

Danny looked up from his flattened ball to see a crowd of people lined up like they were waiting for a parade. Every single person seemed to stare, laugh, and point at him. Danny bolted down the street, his round belly bouncing up and down outside his overstretched T-shirt. Gasping, he stopped to catch his breath and held his chest.

"I hate being fat. I hate being called Chunky Dan! And I really hate having to fight for air—it's scary!" Danny said to himself. "I just wanna have fun like Swish and Carmen—the kinda fun I had before Dad died."

Finally catching his breath, Danny looked up to see the entrance to a gigantic mall that had a Disney World feel. In the parking lot he spotted a humongous bus covered with pictures of kids playing soccer, swimming, riding bikes, and twirling Hula-Hoops. A sign at the entrance read Welcome All Kids—We Make Fitness Fun!

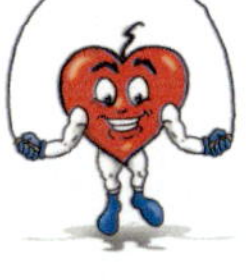

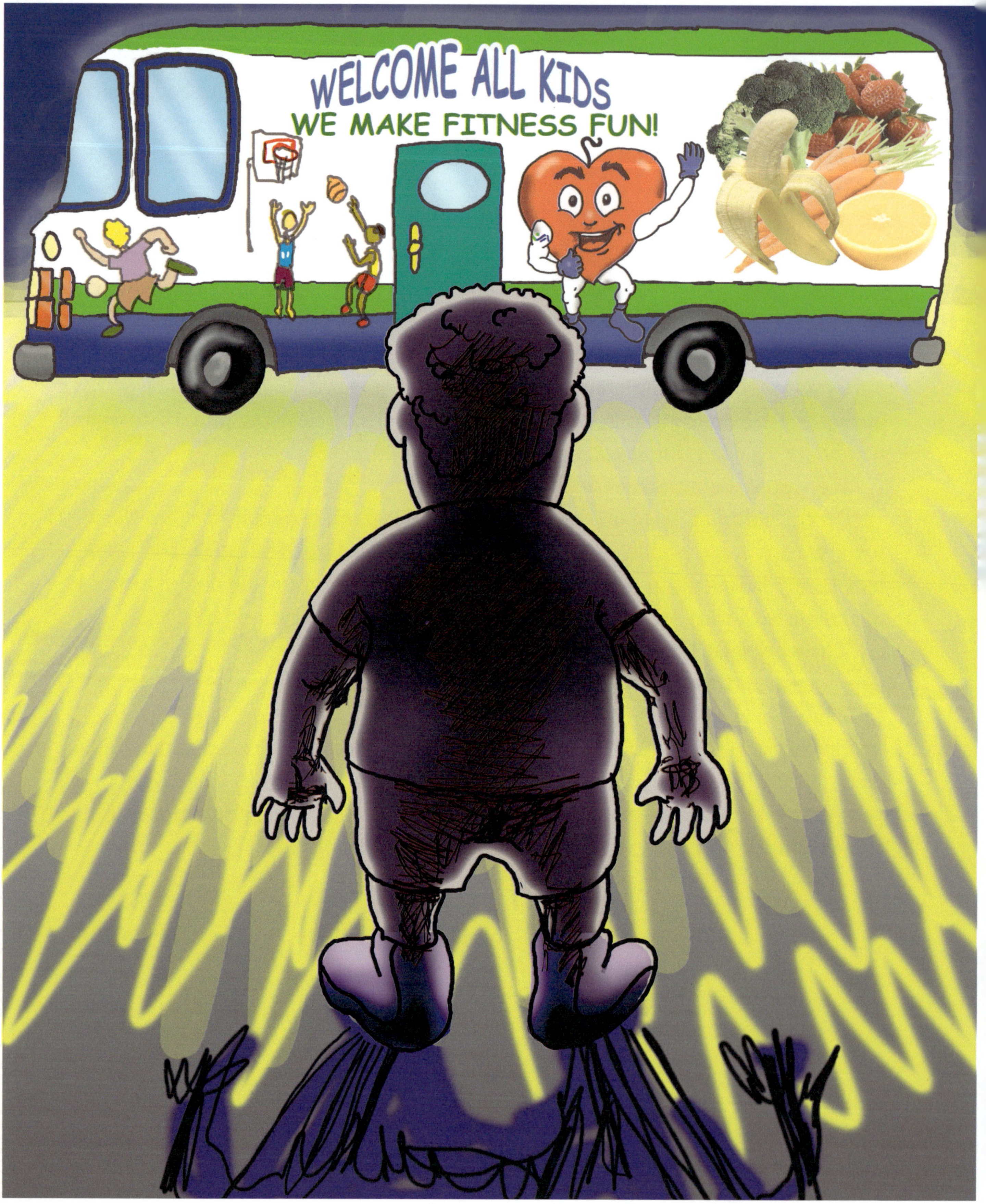
WELCOME ALL KIDS
WE MAKE FITNESS FUN!

"Man, that's the phattest-looking bus I've ever seen! All those kids look so healthy and happy. Maybe this is the answer to my prayers." He looked down at his stomach, grabbed a handful of fat and jiggled it. "I need some belly-be-gone, so I can get back to my old self."

Danny took a long, deep breath, crept up to the bus, and tapped lightly on the door. A smiling, muscular heart with one curly strand of hair sticking straight up opened the door and greeted him. He looked like some kind of superhero from a comic book.

"Hi, I'm the Cardio Kidd, but call me CK. Welcome to the Fit-Mobile!"

"Whoa!" Danny shrieked. He stepped back and rubbed his eyes, "I must be dreaming. Hearts don't talk!"

CK chuckled, and reached out to shake Danny's hand. "See, you're not dreaming."

"Sorry, Mr. CK, I'm Danny Dixon. I didn't mean to be rude, but um, you're the first talking heart I've ever met. I-I-I just can't believe I'm talking with a heart."

"All hearts speak Danny, you just have to listen."

Like a nail being pulled toward a magnet, Danny was drawn inside this magical bus. He poked his head through the door and rolled his eyes up-down-and-side-to-side with a mix of curiosity and excitement.

"WOW! This bus ROCKS, CK! I love these cool shiny-looking bikes with the skinny tires and fancy handlebars. And what's that treadmilly-looking thing with all those wires and a computer on it? What do you do in here? Do you help people lose weight? Can you show me how to get muscles like the boys on the outside of—"

"Slow down, Danny boy. I love your questions!" CK pointed at his chest, "You've got this heart's body pumping with excitement too! In this bus we reach and teach. We help young people reach their unique healthy weight through exercise, and teach them to make healthier food choices."

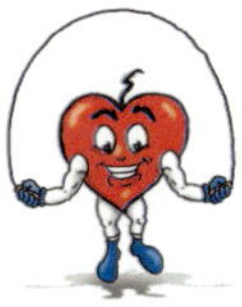

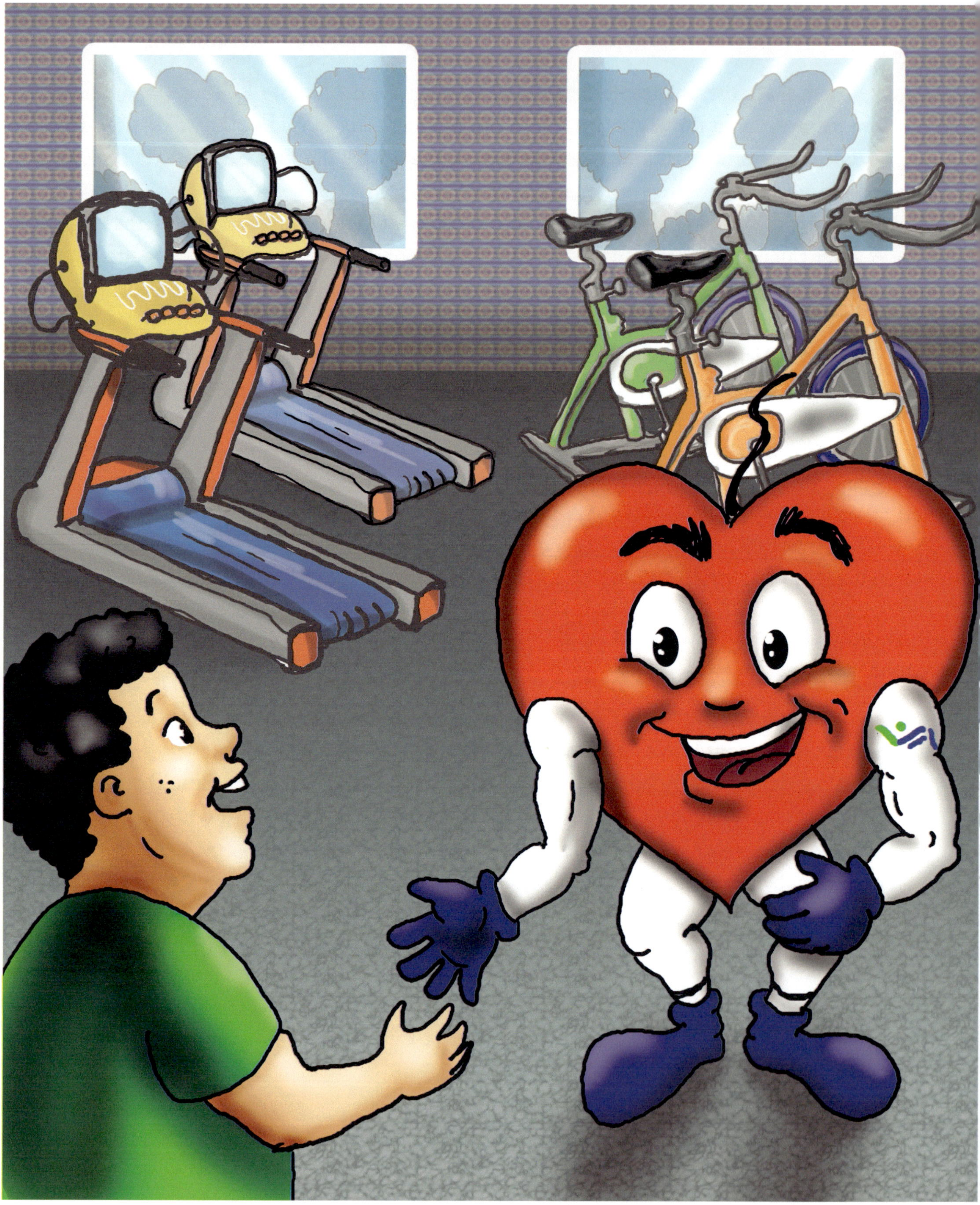

"Great! Cause that's just what I need CK. But uh, what's the cost? I earn fifty-five dollars a month from my part-time job. Only, I spend all of it on cookies, cake, and my favorite—fresh-outta-the-fryer-melt-in-your-mouth glazed doughnuts! But I'd give up anything to look like those kids on the outside of the bus."

CK smiled, "I understand. Sweets are tempting." Then CK got serious and looked the boy straight in the eye. "Okay Danny, here's the real cost. You must pay attention to all the foods you eat. Greasy doughnuts, sugary cookies and fat-filled ice cream are not your friends. They might make you feel good for a hot minute, but I promise you they will only keep you fat and your body unhappy! Your first payment is to become a friend to your body. Choose smart foods like fruits and veggies to make it happy. And you gotta *want* to find them. Are you sure you're ready to pay that kinda price?"

"CK, after the jacked-up day I've had—oh yeah, I'm ready! Danny pumped both fists above his head and boomed, "Let's do it!"

"Then step in and have a seat. So Danny, tell me, why are you so anxious to lose weight?"

"Well CK, I LOVE basketball! My dad was a great college player and taught me to shoot, dribble, pass, rebound, and play defense—everything. I was the best baller in my old neighborhood, and I had a lotta close friends. But last year, one day while we were shooting hoops my dad had a heart attack. By the time the ambulance arrived it was too late. Just before he passed, he squeezed my hand tight and made me promise to keep working on my basketball skills, keep getting good grades and to take care of Mom. But I stopped playing ball because it made me cry to just look at a basketball. Then doughnuts and cookies became my happy pills," Danny sighed.

CK put his arm on Danny's shoulder and said, "I'm very sorry about your dad. That explains a lot."

"Thanks CK. Anyway, my mom thought it would help me if we moved to a new neighborhood, and it sorta worked. I do feel ready to get my game on again—at least in my heart. My body? Well, let's just say the guys think I'm 'too chunky' to be a ballplayer. And to be honest, since gaining this extra weight, I get out of breath way too fast."

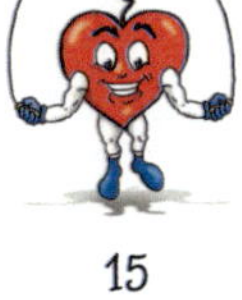

"Don't worry Danny, if you want it badly enough, we'll help you breathe easier, lose weight and get you back on the basketball court."

"We? Who's *we*?"

"You know to be a great basketball player, you need a great team. And I've got the perfect team for you! Meet my FFF!"

Danny snapped his head side-to-side, looking in every corner of the bus. "The FFF?"

CK laughed and opened the refrigerator to reveal a wondrous sight. CK pointed as he introduced his team. "Danny, meet my Fat-Fighting Force. In this corner is Tuffy-McBuffy."

Danny's eyes beamed with a blend of awe and disbelief, as he watched a muscular McIntosh apple pump broccoli spears over his head. Before he could ask a question CK continued, "And over there, the cool and crispy Sista Cellie." She gave Danny a thumbs up while chillaxing on a bed of lettuce, reading Maya Angelou's poetry.

"A poetry-reading celery stalk and a buffed-up apple? This is the bomb bus!"

"And on this shelf Bonita-B, the fabulicious queen of salsa. Check out how she practices her hot tango moves. These healthy fruits and veggies are my Fat-Fighting Force—my FFF," explained CK.

"Yo Danny! Call me T-Mac," McBuffy said. "We heard ya story over our walkie-talkies, and we're gonna help ya bust up this fat that's been dragging you down. I'll help you build muscle by teaching you the right way to lift weights—ya ready to pay that price?"

"I'm ready T-Mac! Danny could already feel his muscles tingling; ready to get his pump on.

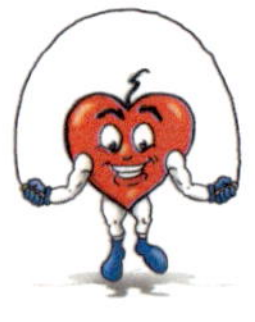

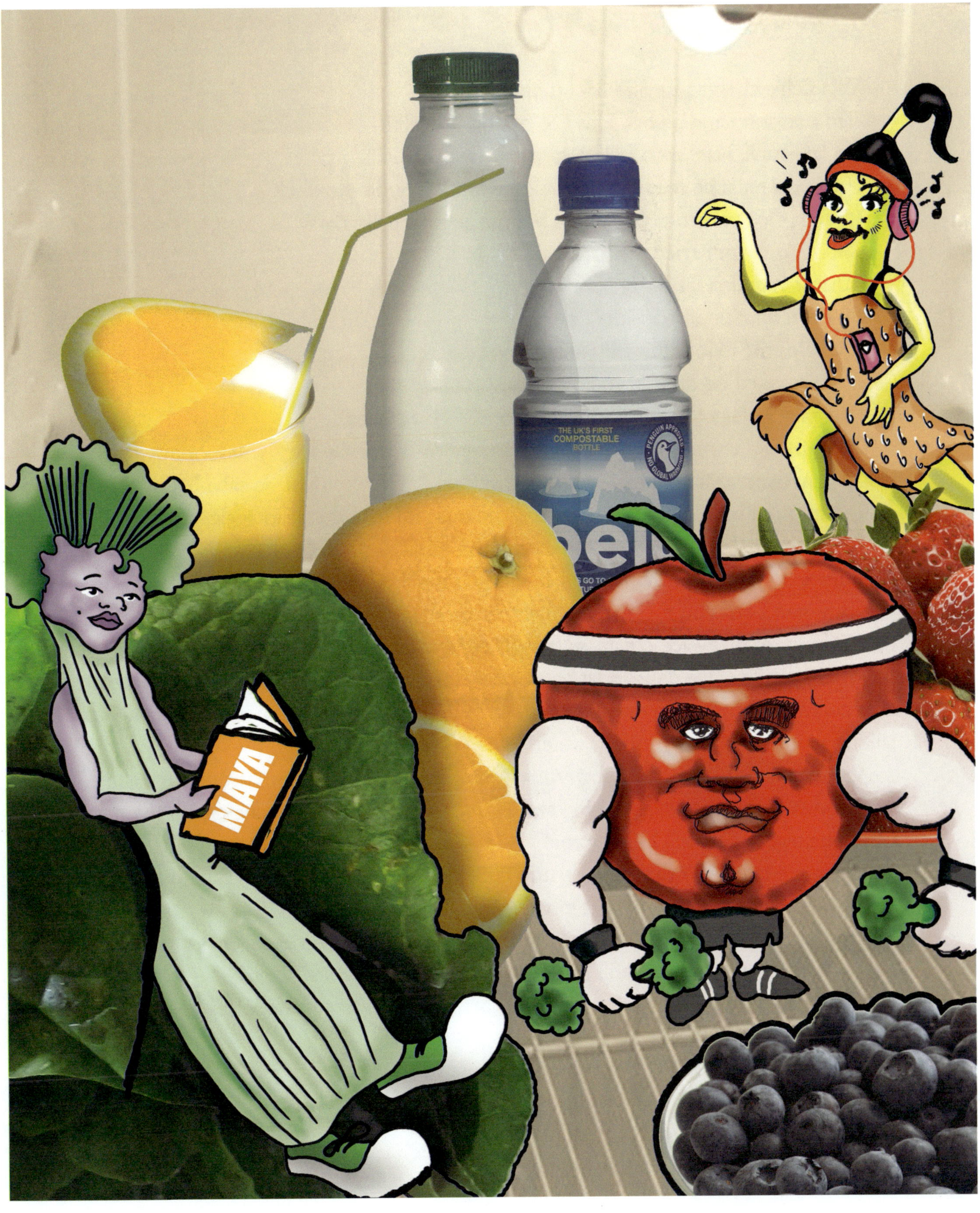
THE UK'S FIRST
COMPOSTABLE
BOTTLE
MAYA

Sista Cellie charged up and fist bumped Danny.

"I'm a sprinter and a poet. I love to rap on the tellie.

I'm laid-back, have zero fat—please call me Sista Cellie.

Now you must be ready to do some sprinting 'round the track.

It's the price you gotta pay if you wanna get that belly flat!"

Then Danny returned the fist bump.

"Yeah, I'm definitely ready Sista Cellie.

I'll even munch on a stalk of celery,

if it helps me to lose this jelly belly!"

Danny poked his middle, and everyone cracked up.

"Hey, the kid's got rhymes and jokes too!" T-Mac ribbed.

"Hola [Hello] Danny! I'm Bonita-B. I loooove to dance the way you loooove to play ball! If you want to have a really fun time getting fit, I'll teach you to salsa."

Danny jumped up and down causing the bus and his tummy to jiggle.

"I can't wait...I've always wanted to learn to salsa!"

"I'll meet you at your house later today, and we'll put together a plan," CK said.

"Hey, can I call you if I get a midnight-snack attack? It's reeeel haaard to sleep when that Chunky Monkey ice cream starts calling my name. While Mom is asleep I tip-toe downstairs and gobble down a fat bowl, along with a dozen or so homemade chocolate chip cookies. Then I wash everything down with two big glasses of ice-cold milk! Just talking about it makes my mouth water!"

CK and Danny laughed. "Call anytime, especially if you get a 'midnight-snack attack.' And always remember this—eating and living healthy is all about choice, it's the price you gotta pay to get back in the game!"

"Thanks a lot CK! With your help and the FFF, I can do this!" Danny high-fived CK as if he had just hit a last-second shot to win a state championship.

Danny watched CK start his daily jog to the park. The heart's single strand of hair whipped and waved behind him like a kite's tail on a windy day.

"Why can't everyone have such a big heart?" he wondered before heading home.

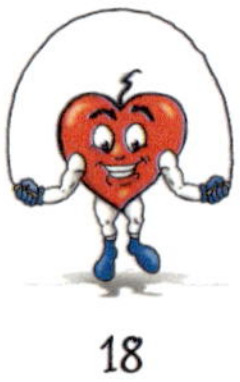

CHAPTER 3:
Getting Back in the Game!

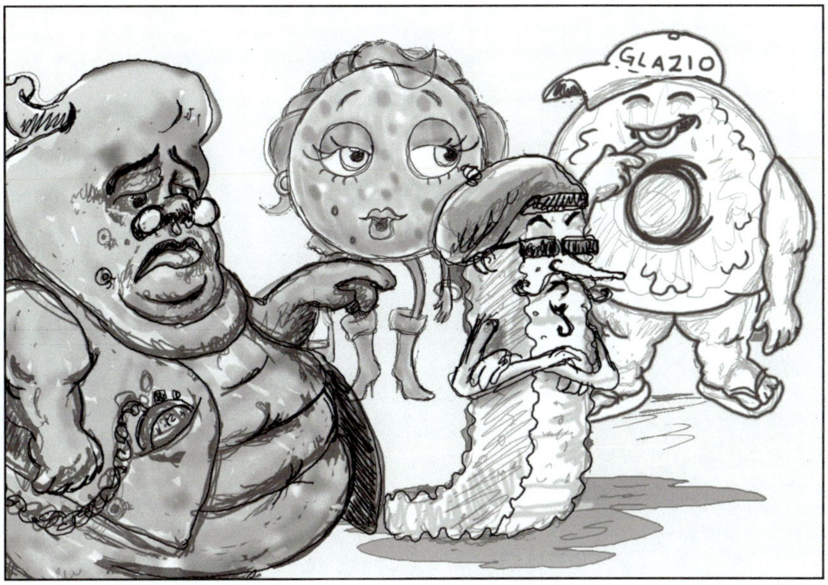

The Blubba Hill Gang Strikes Again!

Though he'd met new friends,
and got his wish,
he'd soon have worse trouble
than being bullied by Swish...

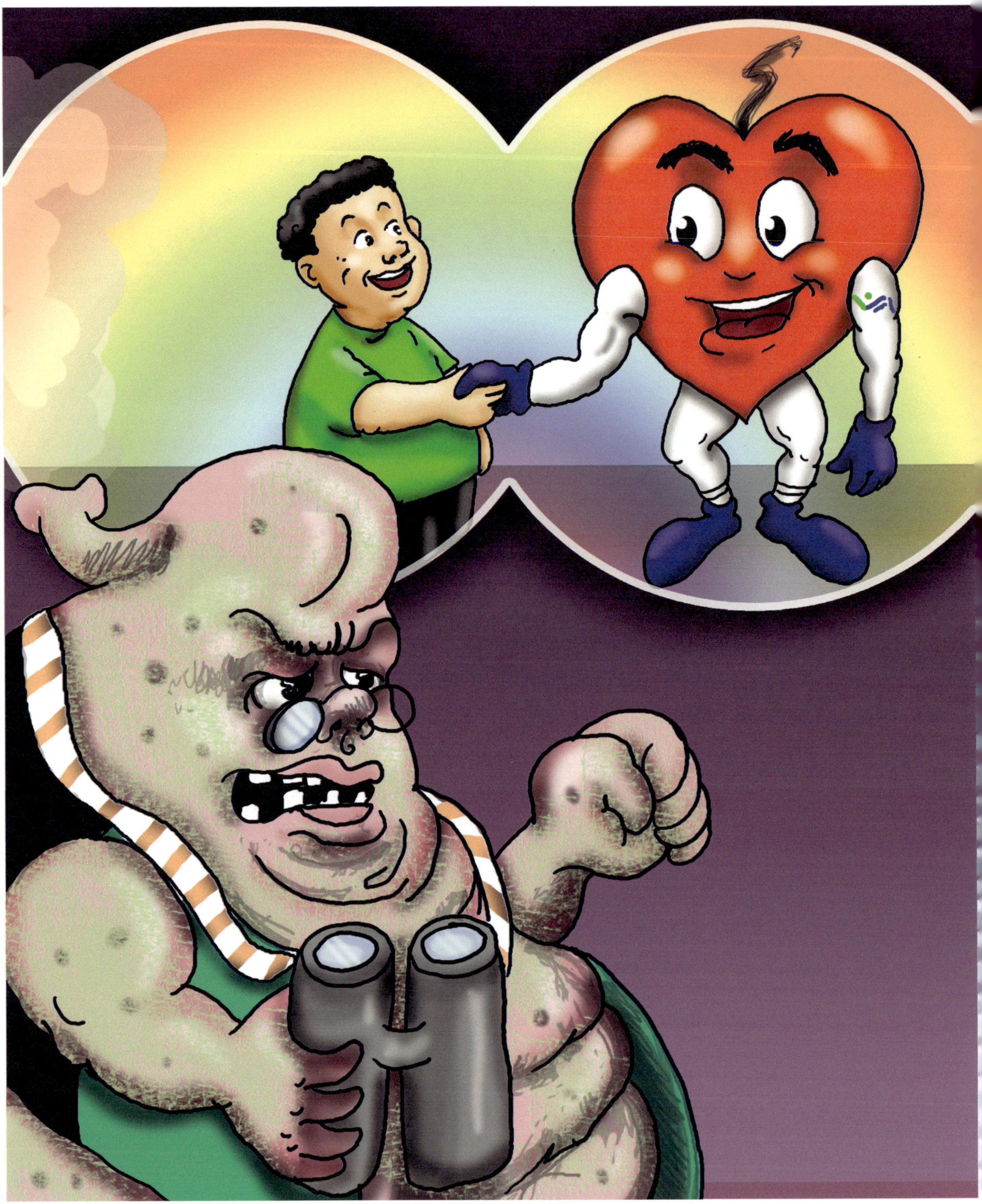

THE BLUBBA HILL GANG STRIKES AGAIN!

While Swish had a mean bark, he had nothing on the notorious Blubba Hill Gang, a crew as cunning as a pack of wild coyotes. They prowled nearby, stalking Danny like a motherless lamb.

Mr. Stuffin-Gutt, the gang's clever ringleader spoke with a high-and-mighty British tone that meant serious business. This greedy, junk-food loving gut's one sinister purpose in life was to create a vast army of chubby, couch-potato kids—or Chunky-Flunkies as he called them.

The gang made a funny sight sneaking along the sidewalk, ducking behind trees so Danny wouldn't see them. Stuffin-Gutt's go-to guy for nasty jobs was Faz-n-Greazy, a slick-talking, crinkled-cut french fry who glided around in his own grease path. When Stuffin-Gutt needed someone to sweet talk a kid into eating sugary foods, Chubbalicious-Chip was his go-to gal. A brassy, sassy, bow-legged chocolate chip cookie, with a heavy "New Yawk" accent, she loved to wear eye-popping red high-heel boots. But even this savvy boss wasn't sure what to make of Sweet Glazio. Yet, he could always depend on his stuttering, lollipop-sucking sidekick to get kids drooling over his powerful freshly fried doughnut aroma.

Danny, new to the neighborhood, had no idea that this gang of tricky junk food peddlers were lurking in the area and were long-time, bitter rivals of the Cardio Kidd and his Fat-Fighting Force. Nor did he realize how sneaky they were at misleading a kid who was on the path to choosing healthy change.

After seeing Danny seemingly float from the Fit-Mobile as if he'd just spent the whole day at Six Flags, Stuffin-Gutt huddled his gang like a football quarterback.

"Listen up Blubbaheads! I've got one flabulously "sweet" plan to catch a new Chunky-Flunky by the nose. Look, we know the One-Haired Wonder gets his snooze-on in his hammock after he runs his sappy heart out. While he's napping, Faz-n-Greazy, I want you to glide up behind him and fill up his insides with plenty of your special heart-clogging grease. That'll give the neighborhood snooper-trooper so much heartburn, he'll be too sick to spoil our Welcome to the Block Sugar Bowl Bash.

"No problem Boss." Faz said. "That snooping, party-pooping heart won't know what hit him!"

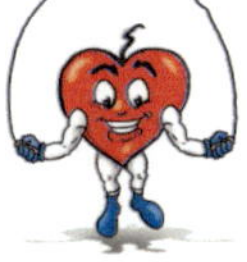

Stuffin-Gutt's voice boomed as he waved his index finger back and forth like a windshield wiper, "Chunky Dan will not, do you hear me...Will NOT get away from us! My belly still aches when I think about how we lost Jelly-Roll Kelly to the Cardio Kidd and his Fat-Fighting Flunkies."

Glazio groaned "Yeah, n-now ol' Jelly-Roll is tr-tr-im and sl-sl-lim. He never dr-dr-drinks soda or eats c-c-andy. We w-wuz r-r-robbed!"

"We WERE robbed Smurf-brain! You really should stop sucking on those Dum-Dum lollipops," Stuffin-Gutt grumbled.

"What's t-that sup-p-pose to m-m-mean, Boss?"

"Never mind Einstein! Once we know Chunky D's top ten 'flavorite' foods, I want you and Chubbalicious-Chip to go junk food shopping. Can you handle that?"

Glazio giggled, "P-p-p-iece of c-c-cake...But you n-need to relax b-b-big fella, you gonna upset your ulsa."

"It's ULCER! AND DON"T TELL ME TO RELAX! Shhhh! Here comes our new Chunky Flunky," Stuffin-Gutt whispered. "Let's follow him home and then put our Sugar Bowl Bash plan into action. Hey, Glazio, turn the power down on your fresh glazed doughnut aroma before Danny gets a whiff. You're making my stomach growl. When we arrive at his house, I'll wink, and then turn it up full blast. I can't wait to see that boy's knees wobble. And he'll need a towel to catch all the drool!"

An Ulcer is a sore in the stomach's lining that's painful and can be made worse by certain food, smoking or stress. Drink plenty of water, eat plenty of high fiber foods and stay chilled.

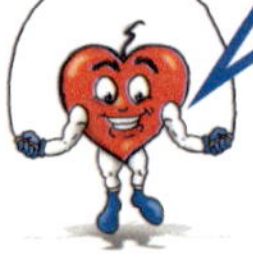

CHAPTER 4:
Getting Back in the Game!

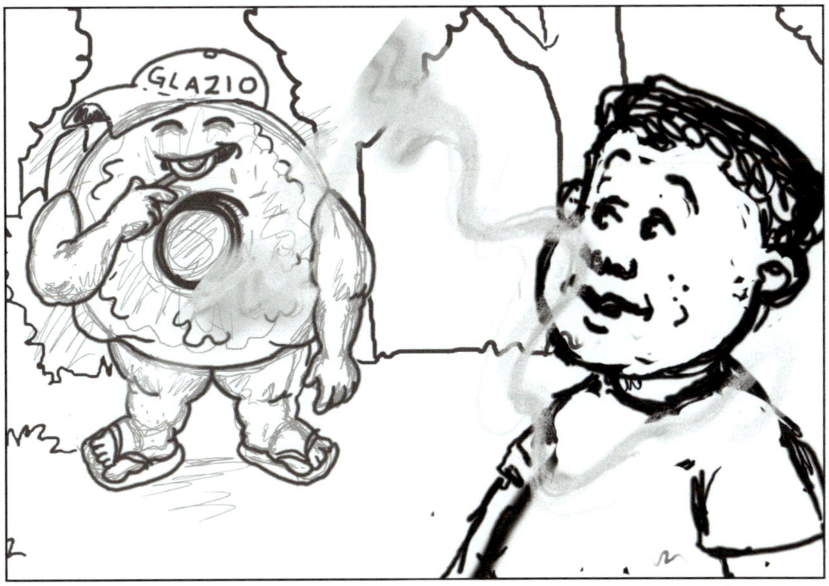

Danny Takes the Bait

The Blubbaheads ducked
in and out bushes
and hid behind cars,
staying just beyond the
view of their prey;
they looked to be from Mars

As Danny turned the key to his front door, he heard what he thought was a motorcycle starting up.

"Excuse me Danny, just clearing my throat. I'm Mr. Stuffin-Gutt, and this is my Blubba Hill Gang."

Danny's eyebrows shot up! He stared Stuffin-Gutt up and down like he was a creature from a sci-fi movie. "Wow," he thought. "Mom won't believe I met a talking heart with one curly strand of hair and a talking stomach wearing a vest, pocket watch, and beat-up bedroom slippers—all in the same day."

The bossy gut snapped his fingers, "Hello, earth to Danny—"

"Hey wait! How did you know my name?"

Stuffin-Gutt pulled out a soiled hankie and wiped the one smudged lens of his horn-rimmed glasses. "Well, we overheard one of the boys at the park call you Chunky Dan. That big bully." He turned and winked at Glazio.

"Now meet my Blubbaheads, starting with my main homefry, Faz-n-Greazy."

Danny didn't know whether to bust out laughing or look for a barf bag when the french fry opened his greasy lips. "Hope he doesn't try to shake my hand," Danny thought.

"Bonjour, Danny boy! I'm slick n' salty, plenty oily, and deep-fried. And I drip a lotta fat-makin' grease everywhere I glide! I'm Faz-n-Greazy!"

"Hey, Mr. Faz, no disrespect, but would you mind putting a freeze on that grease and not dripping it in front of my house?"

"No worries," Faz said.

"Hmmm, next time I'm in a restaurant I think I'll pass on the fries and choose coleslaw," Danny mumbled under his breath.

A bow-legged cookie with red, thigh-high boots pushed Faz aside. "Hmmm, at least she's got cute dimples," Danny mused.

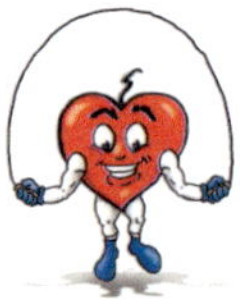

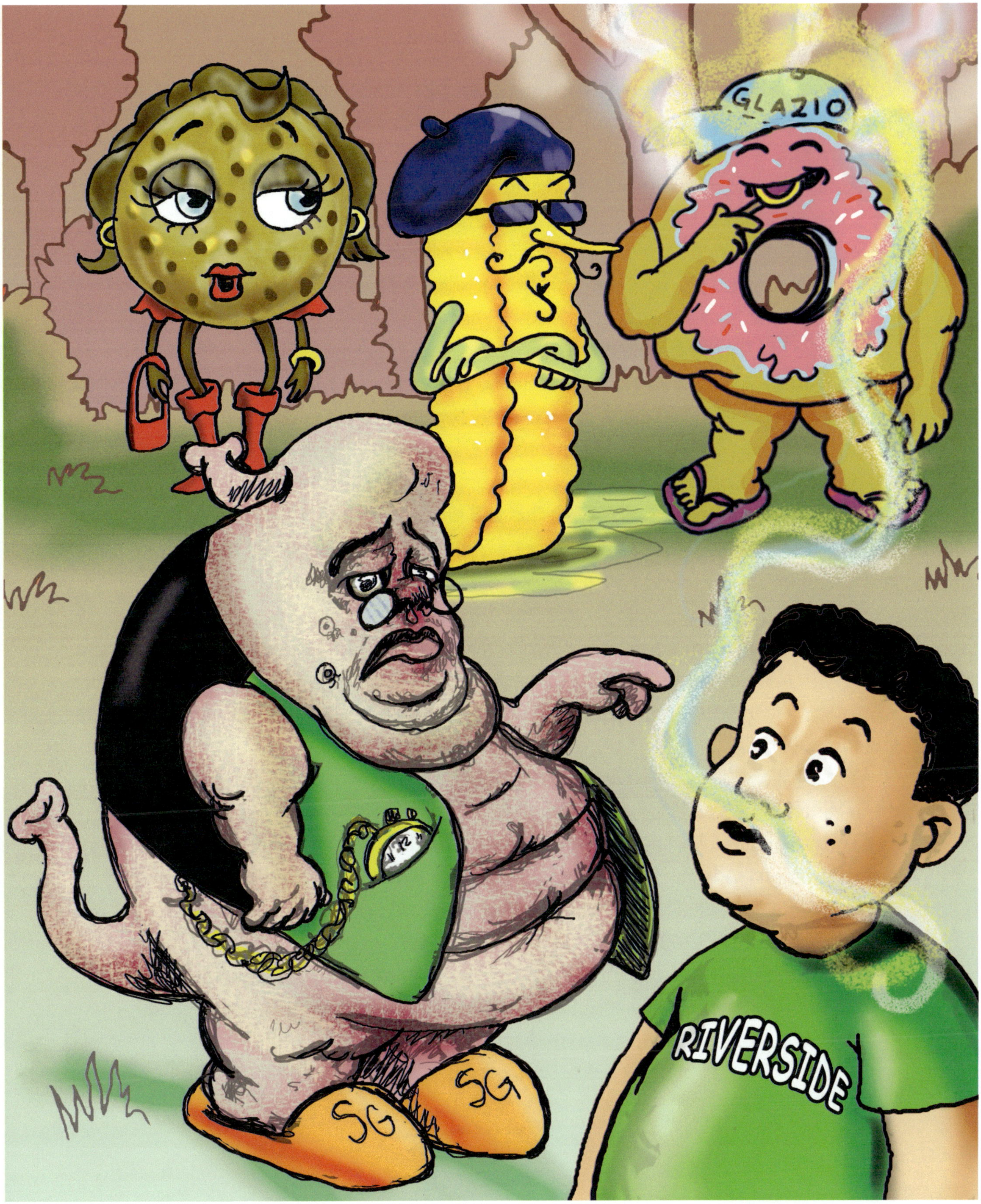
GLAZIO
SG
SG
RIVERSIDE

"Hubba-hubba, this chubby cookie packs plenny-a-shuga and may not be that nutritious. But I'm sho 'nuff a ton-a-fun to eat—that's why they call me Chubbalicious, the Hip Chip!"

"Ahhh..., it suddenly smells like a glazed doughnut bakery out here!" Danny said. "Let me guess, that's your lollipop-sucking doughnut friend over there."

Stuffin-Gutt swiped a clump of Glazio's sweet coating and licked his fingers clean. "You're right. That is the one and only Sweet Glazio! Doesn't his fresh doughnut aroma make your taste buds juicy?"

An excited Danny smacked his lips, "Heck, yeah!"

"M-m-making people f-f-fat and h-h-happy is my claim to f-f-fame. I'm a d-d-ee-licious doughnut; Sweet Gl-Gl-Glazio is my name. Ni-Nice to meet you Danny!"

Entranced by Glazio's hypnotic aroma, all Danny could think about was wrapping his lips around that doughnut's sugary glaze. After he felt Danny bite the bait, Stuffin-Gutt continued to reel Danny in like a fish that had given up the fight.

"We saw you on the basketball court earlier today, and we were most upset about how those mean boys dissed you. I know your feelings were hurt."

Danny nodded, "Yes, I was hurt at first, but I met—"

"So we thought up a yummy way to chase your blues away Danny, we want to throw you a Welcome to the Block Sugar Bowl Bash—and guess what? We're bringing all your *fla-vor-ite* sweet treats, including fresh-outta-the-fryer-melt-in-your-mouth glazed doughnuts!"

"Yessss! Warm glazed doughnuts are my flavorite! How did you know?"

"UMMM, LUCKY GUESS!" they said all together.

Danny scratched his head, "Hmmm, a Sugar Bowl Bash sounds very tempting. Only I just met new friends, the Cardio Kidd and his FFF. And they're going to help me change my unhealthy food choices, so I can lose this jelly-belly, get healthier, and feel better. But best of all, I'll get back to basketball—the game I love! "

A smirking Chubbalicious Chip batted her long, thick eyelashes and quipped,

"Uh-huh, we know al-l-l-l about Mr. Tell-everybody-how-to-live Cardio Kidd."

"Hey, Chubbalicious! Don't diss my friend—"

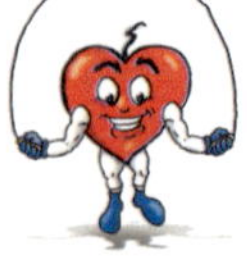

"Look, Danny, the Kidd and his FFF tawk a great game, but that's all it is—TAWK!"

Faz-n-Greazy tipped down his dark sunglasses, stuck out his tongue, and said, "Yuk! What cool kid wants to eat stringy celery sticks, runny tomatoes and hard-to-chew apples after a looooong hard day sitting in class?"

"But—"

"But nothing!" Stuffin-Gutt snapped. "Here Danny boy, jot down your top ten flavorite fun foods—your FFF."

Danny took the pad and pen, paused and shook his head, remembering..."Wait, FFF is CK's crew, and it stands for Fat-Fighting Force."

Stuffin-Gutt took another thick swipe of Glazio's sweet coating and held it right under Danny's nose. "Now really, which would you prefer, tasteless celery sticks or this? Good! We'll meet you in one hour, so please don't munch and spoil your appetite, okay?"

Danny wanted to say no, but his hand seemed to have a mind of its own as it scribbled ten of his favorite foods. Danny dragged himself inside like a car rolling on four flat tires. He flipped on his Xbox, but quickly flipped it off, stood up, and looked long and hard at himself in the mirror.

Licking his lips like the ol' sly fox that just swallowed the rabbit, Stuffin-Gutt gloated, "Way to go my blubba-lovin', artery-clogging friends! Did you see Chunky Dan's knees buckle when I put Glazio's sweet coating under his nose?"

"Yeah Boss. And his mouth puffed up like a baby guppy waiting to be fed a worm!" Chubba-Chip cracked. The Blubbaheads cackled like a coop full of hens.

"Now let's give our new Chunky-Flunky a Sugar Bowl Bash he'll never forget."

An artery is a tube that carries blood from your heart to your cells and other vital organs. When it gets clogged, your heart must work harder to do its job, and wears out faster. Be smart with your heart—eat healthy!

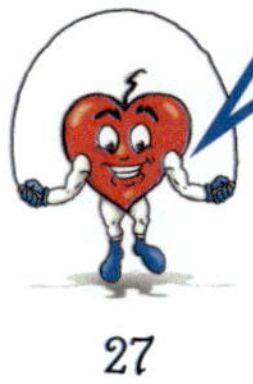

CHAPTER 5:
Getting Back in the Game!

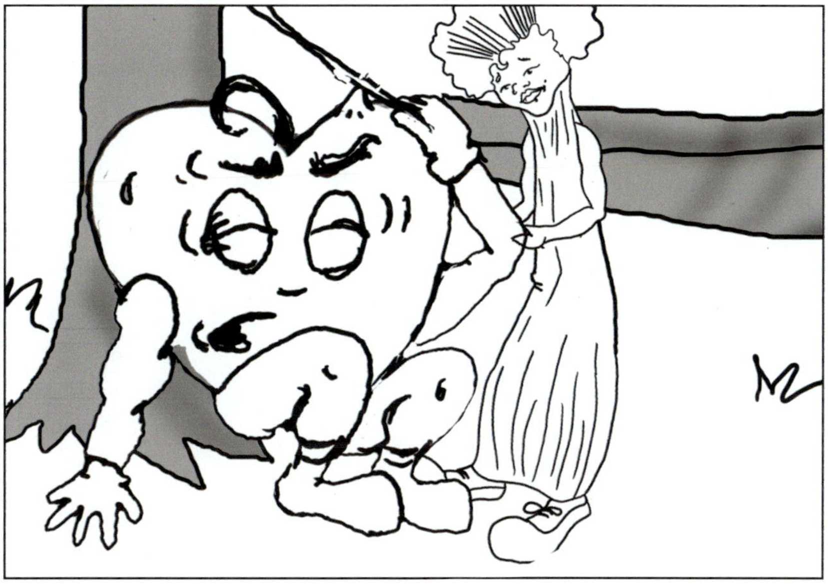

The Cardio Kidd Goes Down

As CK napped in the park,
he was a happy heart at peace
But Faz came from nowhere
and filled him up with fatty grease!

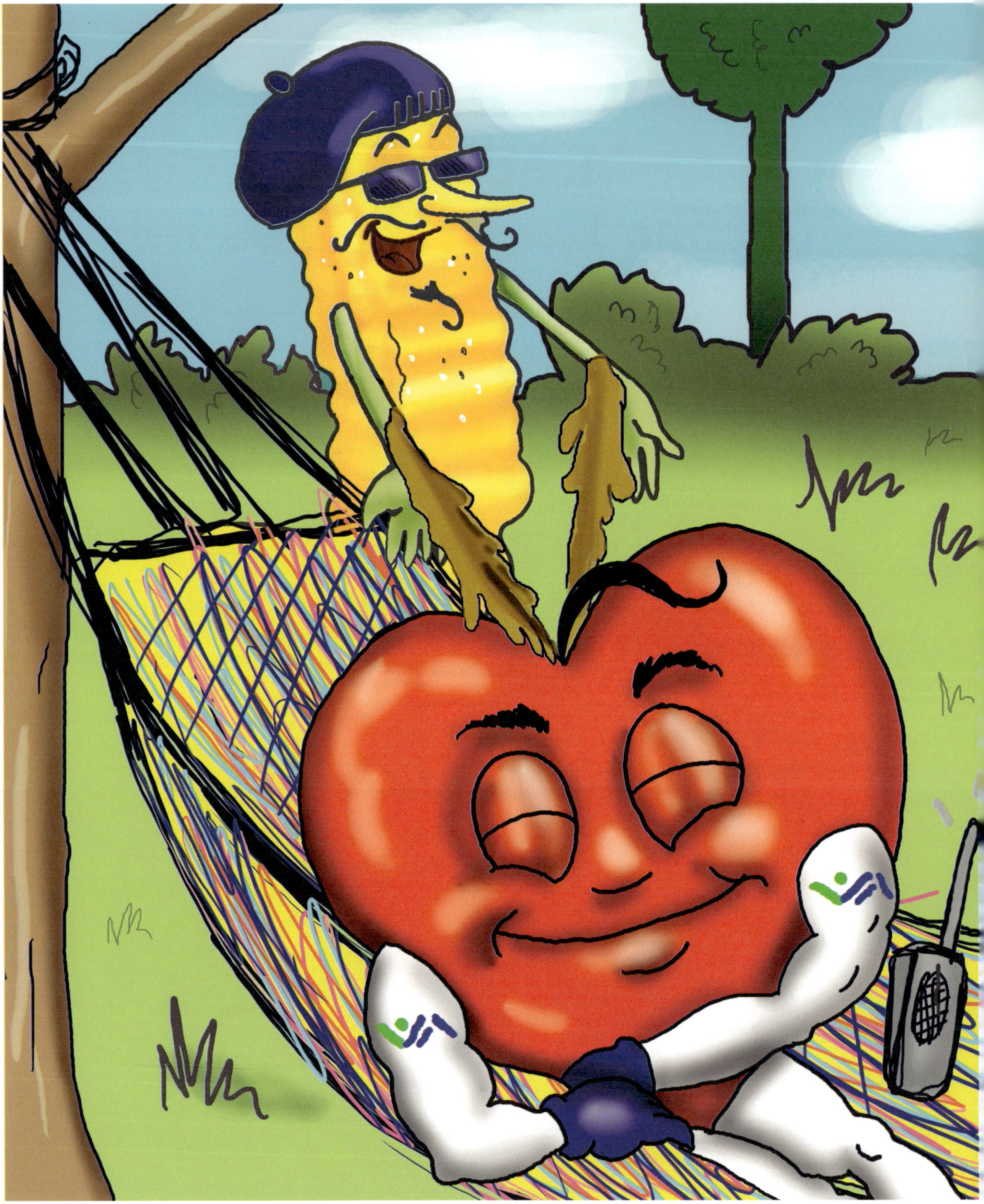

Using the automatic grease-releaser in his wrist, Faz sprayed CK's insides with his special heart-clogging, greasy sludge. "Take THIS Cardio Kidd!"

In a heartbeat CK's head began spinning like an out of control merry-go-round. He plopped to the ground and bumped his head.

The brave heart tried to stand but staggered and fell. He fumbled around for the emergency call button on his walkie-talkie. His trembling finger barely had the strength to send a distress signal to his FFF. Sista Cellie, practicing for a poetry slam, saw the flashing red light on her walkie-talkie.

"Hey guys! CK's in a serious jam and you know who's behind it. Chop-chop! Let's rock!"

The FFF sprang into action like well-trained firemen preparing to battle a fire. They quickly filled their water blasters and water balloons, stuck them into their backpacks and sprinted to the park. Sista Cellie and Bonita-B led the way, their curly hair flying behind them, while stumpy-legged Tuffy-McBuffy struggled to keep up. They found a dizzy CK slumped against a tree; his single power hair was flopped over between his beet-red eyes like an overcooked noodle. Next to CK an exhausted Faz was laid out on the ground; spraying all that grease had zapped him of his strength.

"Oh no, the FFF is here with water blasters!" A pooped-out Faz hopped up and glided out of the park just before being soaked by the FFF's water blasters, leaving a trail of grease puddles behind him.

"Hurry...Flush out this slimy sludge" CK moaned.

Sista Cellie and Bonita-B aimed their water blasters at the top of his head and began flushing CK with fresh water; after a few minutes he was pumping stronger.

Bonita-B whooped, "Look, his power hair is rising! Ahhh...The Kidd is back!"

T-Mac reached out his steely arm and helped CK to his feet.

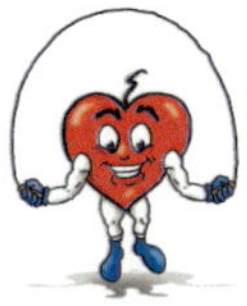

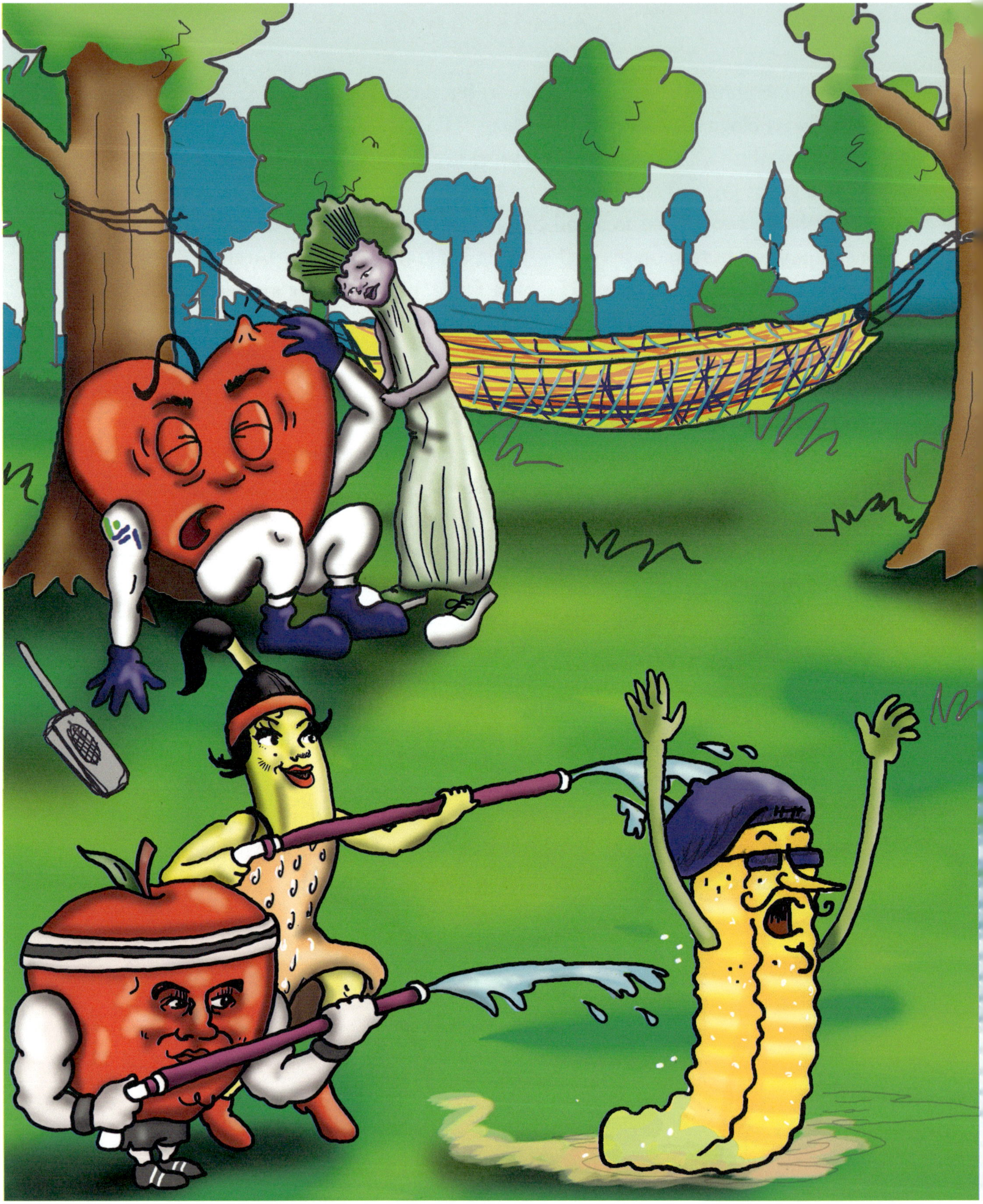

"Thanks, T-Mac! You guys are lifesavers. Now we need to save Danny from the Blubbaheads. Bonita-B, are you ready to serve your special Banana Slip-n-Slide Surprise?"

"Si mi amigo [Yes, my friend]!"

"Bueno [Good]!" CK replied.

"T-Mac, how's our water supply?"

"It's all good, CK!"

The FFF lined up side-by-side and their fired-up leader looked his team in the eye and gave each of them a double fist bump. "C'mon, let's teach Jabba-the-Gutt and his greasy junk food mob a lesson," CK said.

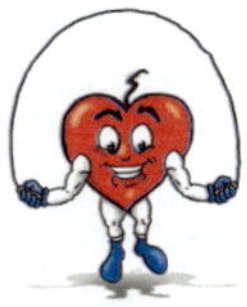

CHAPTER 6:
Getting Back in the Game!

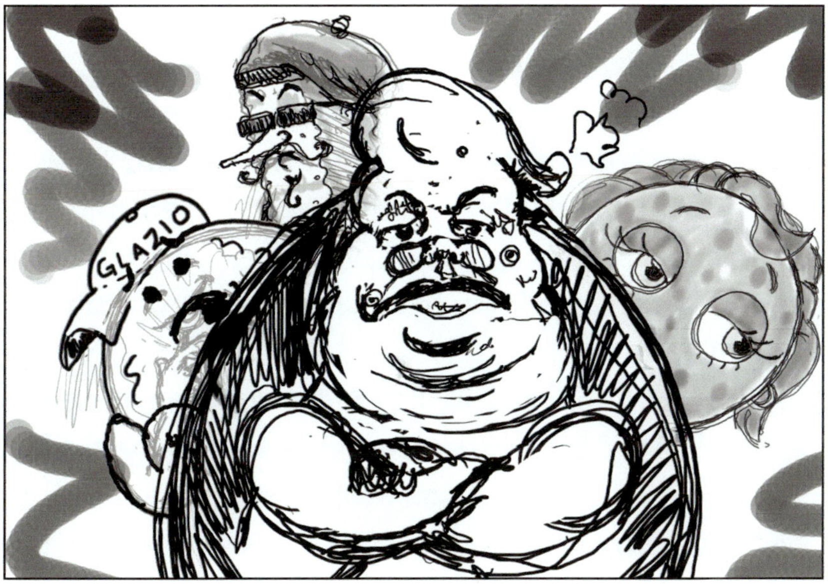

It's a Sugar Bowl Bash & Surprise Water Clash!

*It's tough to make
healthy food choices every day.
If you slip and fall, getting back up
is the price you must pay.*

"*Ummmmm!*" moaned Chubbalicious-Chip. "These warm, moist glazed doughnuts are toe-curling dee-licious! Here Danny, grab a handful, they'll take your taste buds on a mouthwatering joyride."

"Okay, but one 'mouthwatering joyride' is enough or I'll never slim down and get back in the game." Danny took one bite—and poof! The doughnut vanished.

"Well Danny," Mr. Stuffin-Gutt jabbed. "If CK and his so-called Fat-Fighters were true friends, they would have given you a welcome to the block bash, right?"

Danny didn't answer right away because his tongue was too busy swiping every bit of the doughnut's sugary glaze from around his lips and fingers.

"I guess so—I mean no! Look, you did bring all my fav sweets, so I don't want to hurt your feelings by not eating your food. But I'm sick of being too heavy. Look at this, I wear holes in my pants 'cause my thighs rub together, and when I walk a long distance I get blisters. When my mom takes me out, I have to wear clown-looking stretchy pants. It's embarrassing, man. And when I play ball, I breathe so hard, I can't even run halfway up the court without—"

"Reeeelax, my friend. This is a special, fun-to-the-last-crumb celebration," the sweet-talking Chubbalicious chimed in. "Besides, everybody knows you CAN'T have a Sugar Bowl Bash without fun food like ice cream, cookies, cake, and sugary cola to wash it all down, right? And how many kids you know get a special party like this?"

"Well, I guess, but..."

"Don't fight the feeling Danny. Now close your eyes and open wide for Chubbalicious. Here, gobble down this super-gooey, nice n' chewy chocolate chip cookie." She jammed the whole cookie in his mouth. "Good job! I'm so proud of you Danny!"

"Hey Glazio! Get our new friend a King Kong size bowl of Chunky Monkey ice cream, and dress it up real pretty with sweet and colorful sprinkles."

Danny's eyes lit up at the thought of feasting on his fav ice cream.

"G-g-great idea b-b-boss!"

Mr. Stuffin-Gutt pushed his horn-rimmed glasses up the bridge of his nose, checked his watch, and winced, "Hey guys, my stomach is feeling kinda *queasy*."

"Maybe it's the two ga-ga-gallons of i-i-ice cream, dozen d-d-doughnuts and..."

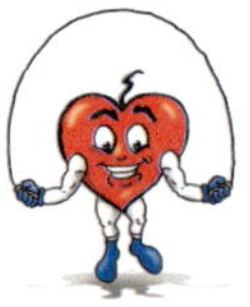

"Put a sock in it Glazio! I'm worried about Faz. He should have been back by now. Give him a call."

"Sorry b-boss, my b--b-battery is dead, and y-y-ou know I d-don't wear s-s-socks."

"Your battery is always dead, just like that lonely brain cell in your fluffy head."

Chubbalicious's cell phone rang. "Is that you, Faz? Where are you? Why are you huffing and puffing?"

"I need...help. Now! I'm about...t-t-two, three...blocks...away from...Chunky D's house. Hurry!"

"What's wrong with Faz?" asked Stuffin-Gutt.

"He sounds woozy. If you ask me ol' Frenchy's been deep fried one too many times. Let's roll. He's right down the street."

Stuffin-Gutt turned to Danny, "Hey big fella, we need to step out for a few minutes and check on Faz. Meanwhile, keep cranking those jaws—you still have plenty more stacks of sweet goodies to gobble up."

The Blubbaheads waddled along the sidewalk in a single file. When they found Greazy, their spuddy was sprawled over a mailbox, drenched in oily sweat, and breathing heavily.

"Oh my word! What happened Faz?"

"I...I...I sprayed my heart-clogging grease...inside CK like you told me, and he...he got sick...and...uh...a short time later his FFF showed up with wa—"

Queasy is a sick or upset feeling in your stomach. It usually happens when you eat too much food.

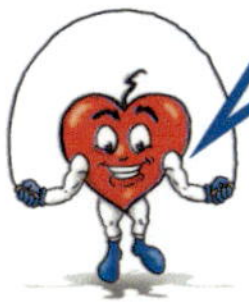

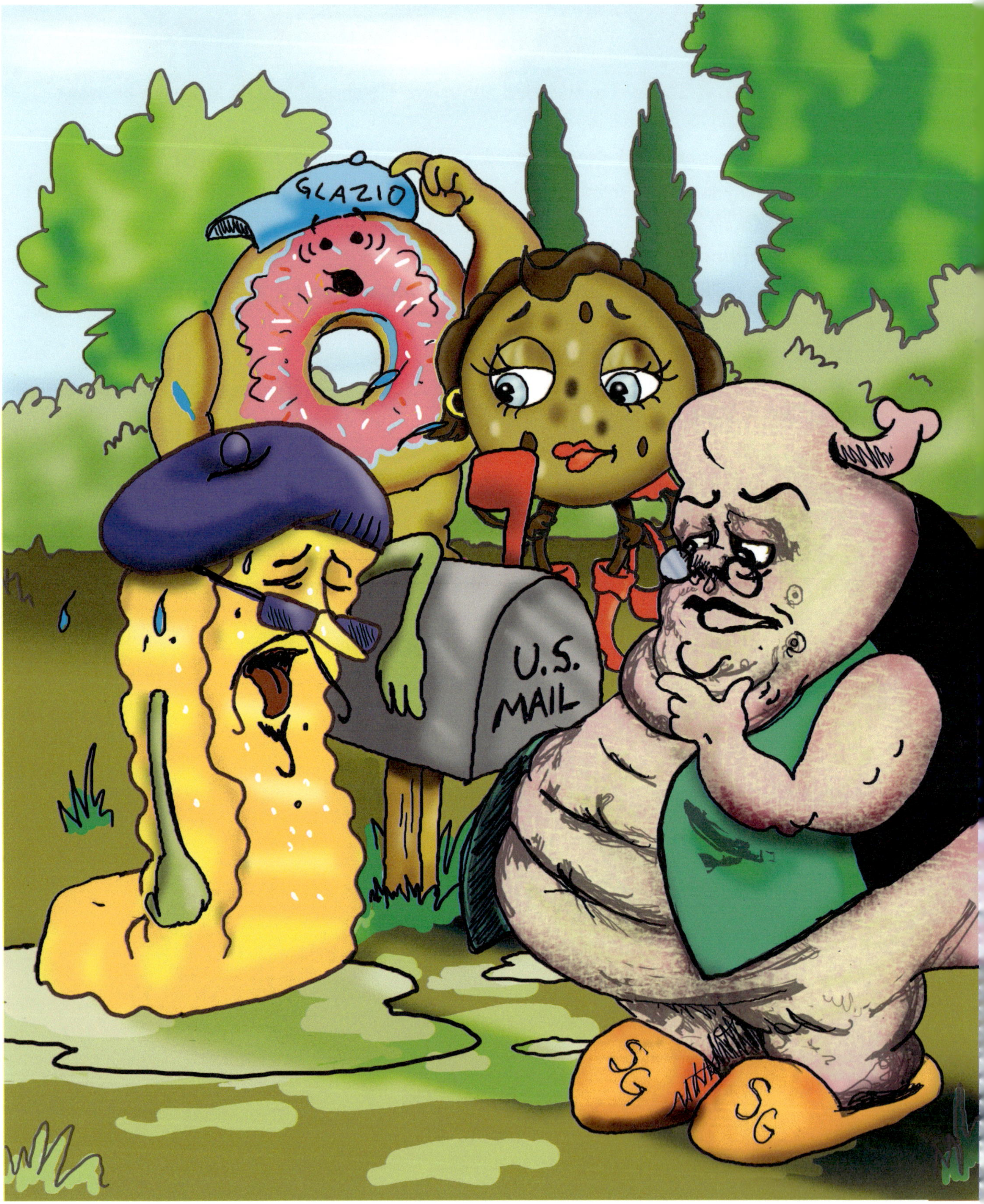
GLAZIO
U.S. MAIL
SG
SG

"Save your breath! We've got to stop those Sugar Bowl Bashing crashers, or they'll brainwash Chunky D into eating healthy and exercising."

"Hey B-b-boss?" asked the ditzy doughnut, "How do you wa-wash b-b-brains?"

"You're bloomin' hopeless, Glazio. Let's head back to Danny's house and plan our next move."

"Dang, my belly feels like it's going to bust open." Suddenly Danny's eyes were drawn to the picture of him and his Dad playing ball together. He abruptly stopped chomping on a glazed doughnut. Then his eyes swept across the family room; he was totally surrounded by stacks of half-eaten sugary sweets—sweets he barely recalled eating. Danny said out loud, "Look at this mess! Please, let this be a bad dream."

But Danny knew this was no dream...Cookie crumbs, potato chips, and sugary glaze were scattered all over the floor. There wasn't a part of the kitchen table or counters that weren't covered with pizza crusts, candy wrappers, drippy ice cream containers, or open soda cans. Then he heard CK's words ringing in his ears, "Remember, eating and living healthy is all about choice!" Danny charged toward the garbage can, kicking a whole box of glazed doughnuts and sending them flying through the air. He spat out the half-chewed doughnut and yelled, "ENOUGH! I'm letting my friend CK down. I'm letting my mom and dad down. But most of all, eating this unhealthy junk is letting my body down!"

Danny knew what he had to do. He grabbed his cell phone and dialed. "CK, this is Danny. I messed up and let Stuffin-Gutt and his Blubbaheads give me a Sugar Bowl Bash. There's junk food EVERYWHERE! I'm so angry with myself for falling for their trickery. They're down the street right now checking on Faz, but they'll be back soon. What should I do?"

"Take a deep breath. It's going to be okay Danny. Everyday you'll be challenged to make healthy food choices, and sometimes you may fall short. You did the right thing by reaching out. Okay, tell the Blubbaheads that your mom is coming home soon, and you need help cleaning the house. They'll scatter faster than sprayed roaches because they're allergic to work. And when the bums rush out the door, they'll get the soggiest slip-n-slide-surprise of their lives."

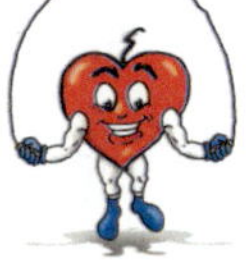

"Okay CK, gotta run. I feel the floor shaking—Big Foot is coming."

The Blubba Hill Gang marched right in without ringing Danny's bell. After eyeballing every part of the room, Stuffin-Gutt's face looked like he'd just been stung by a swarm of wasps. He dipped his head and peered at Danny above his glasses.

"Hmmm...It appears you haven't eaten diddley squat since we left. What have you been doing, mate?"

"Well, my mom will be home soon, and I had to start cleaning up this mess before she walks through that door. Can I count on my new friends to help?"

Stuffin-Gutt glanced down at his pocket watch and cleared his throat, "Ahem! Sorry Dan, we'd love to, but...um...we're already late for Sweet-Tooth Sarah's Sugar Bowl Bash, and we need to get more jun—. Uh, we need to get more fun foods. See ya!"

The whole gang dashed for the door and tried to squeeze through at the same time. But Faz got sandwiched between Stuffin-Gutt and Glazio.

"Hey, you two are squeezing the grease outta me!" Stuffin-Gutt bullied through first but slipped hard to the ground, losing his spectacles. Faz glided out next, followed by Glazio and Chubbalicious, all falling over themselves to make a quick exit.

"Hey, s-somebody dropped ba-ba-nana p-p-peelings all over the pl-pl—"

"Duh! It's a trap! Help me up!" yelped Stuffin-Gutt.

"Where can we get a crane?"

"Not funny, Greazy."

All the Blubbaheads tugged and pulled until Stuffin-Gutt was on his feet. He brushed himself off, gritted his few remaining teeth, and then growled, "All right, I've had it up to my gullet with you Sugar-Bowl-Bash crashers!"

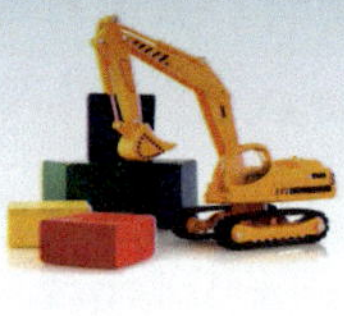

Cranes are used to lift heavy objects, especially on building sites.

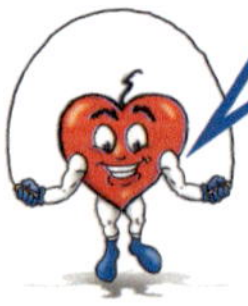

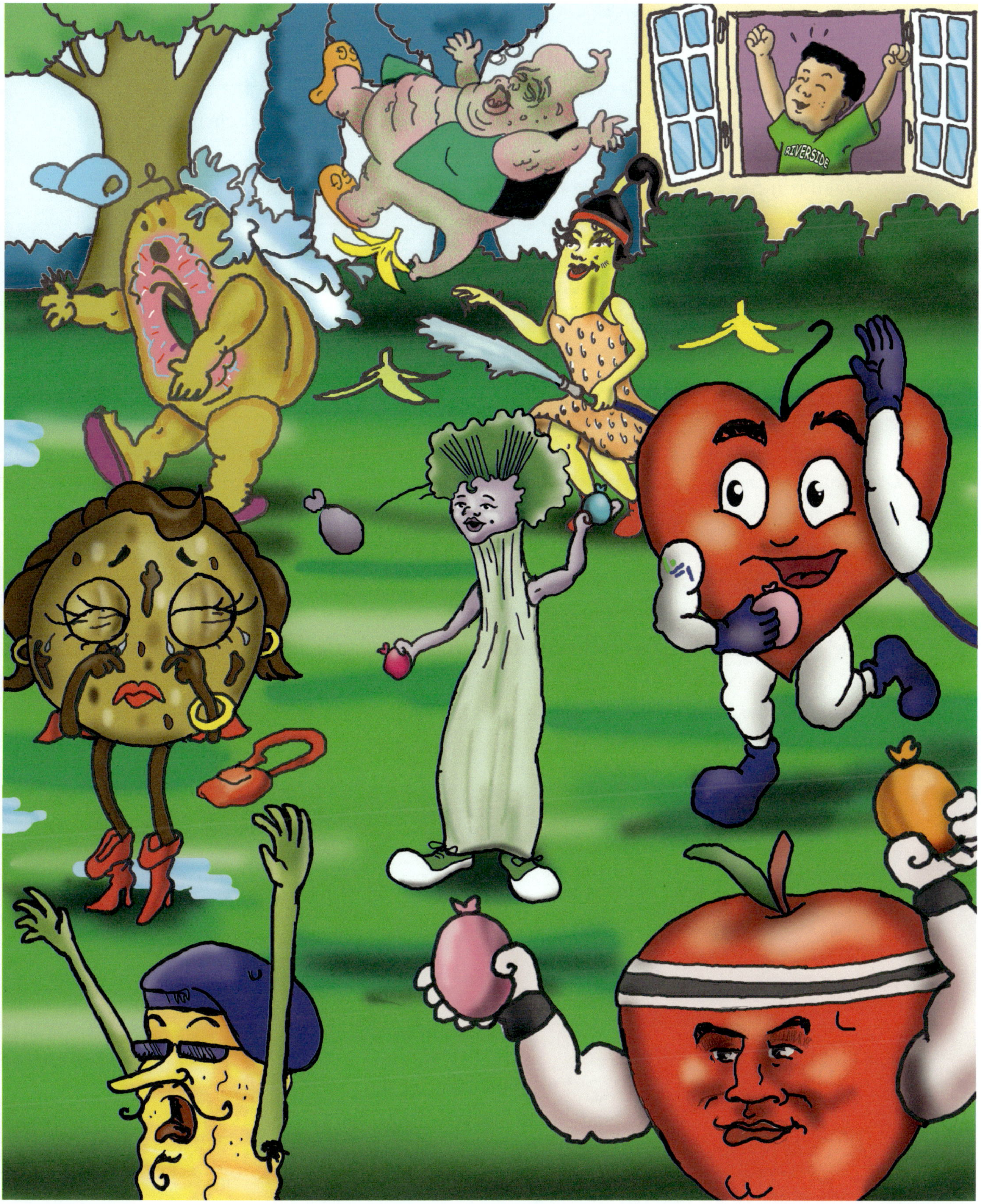
RIVERSIDE

Glazio suddenly raised his arms, "W-w-watch out! It's a w-w-w-ater balloon!" Spladow! "Yessss Bonita-B! Way to dunk on that glazy doughnut!" Danny cheered from his window.

"Ohhh n-n-no! My sugarcoating is m-m-m-elting," sobbed Glazio.

"And my chocolate chips are dripping—look out! They've got water blasters too! Let's get outta here before we all turn to mush!" screamed Chubbalicious.

Stuffin-Gutt stomped his feet, pumped his fists, and roared, "Where's your Blubbahead pride! Don't scurry for the hills like a pack of squeaking, spineless rats! Get back here right now!"

Faz pointed toward Stuffin-Gutt, "Hey guys, we can't leave the big fella all alone. He'll get sprayed down with their water blasters."

"Hey Faz, between you and me, the big fella could use a total body spray-down." Chubbalicious scrunched her nose, "Have you smelled that mad funk under his armpits lately? I think some critter has crawled up there and died. Besides, you know none of us can take a chance on getting wet."

"You're right," Faz nodded his head. "But he's our leader. I tell you what, let's stand behind him, this way we'll all stay dry."

The bleary-eyed Blubbaheads turned around and shuffled back to Danny's front yard. *SQUISH!—SQUISH!—SQUISH!* "What's that n-n-noise?"

"My n-n-new boots!! They're RUINED!" cried Chubbalicious. "This is just all wrong."

While his soggy friends shivered in fear behind him, Stuffin-Gutt fiercely stood his ground.

"What's he doing?" every member of the FFF asked CK in unison. To their amazement Stuffin-Gutt swept his hands in wide circles and began spitting out a rap:

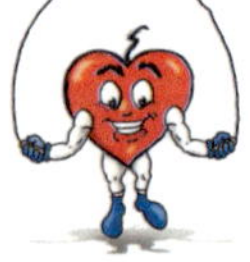

"You really think I'm afraid of a little water spray?
I need a cool shower, it's been a long hot day.
I'm the junk food king, a sugar-loving tubby,
my joy in life is helping kids get chubby.
Gimme plenty pop and a bowl of greasy chips,
sugar cookies and cake keep me licking my lips.
Fruits and veggies—so boring! No fun to eat,
you chase away fat—taste blaze! Not sweet.
Running and jumping ought to be made a crime;
sleeping and eating are MY *sweetest* pastimes.
Who wants tight muscles or a tummy that's flat?
Who wants to lift weights and eat no yummy fat?
Yes, I've got three chins, and my teeth have holes,
haven't seen my toes lately and gotta belly full of rolls.
But ENOUGH talk of bird food and teaching kids to get fit.
This town is too small—one of us must leave lickety-split.
So take your best shot, I dare you to try,
I'll huff and puff and blow you right to the sky! HA-HA-HA!"

Mr. Stuffin-Gutt crossed his stubby arms, puffed up his saggy chest, pulled down his horn-rimmed specs and stared down the FFF.

"Oh really? Hey guys, should we whip out the veggie juice for Mr. *Tuff*-n-Gutt?" asked CK.

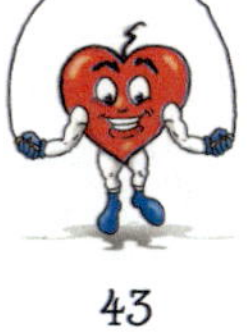

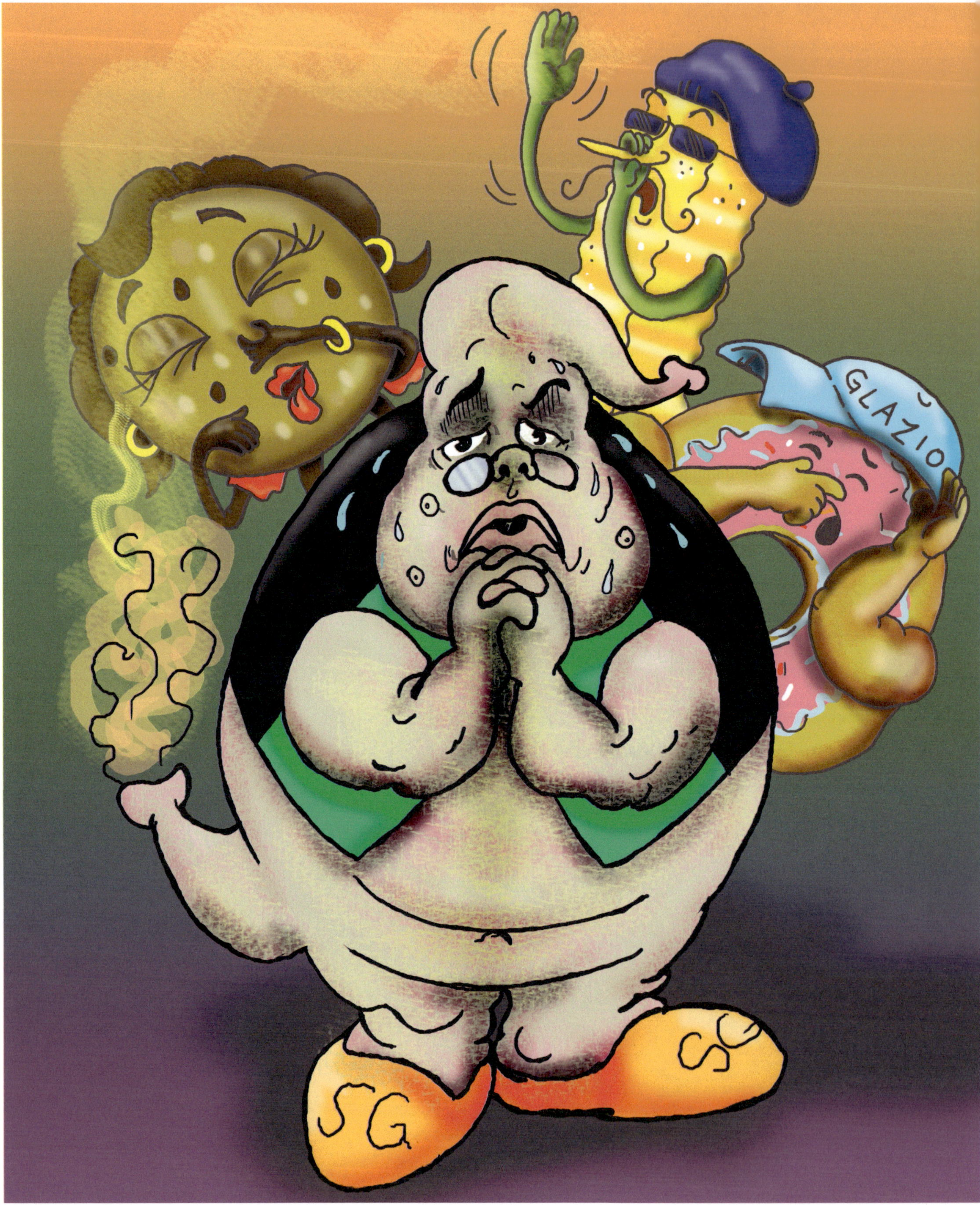
GLAZIO
SG
SG

"The w-w-what?" Stuffin-Gutt stammered. "Oh now wait, CK. Have a heart old pal, old chum. Pl-please...no v-veggie juice! Just one whiff of that low-fatty, tomato-ee smelling stuff, and there'll be a BIG stinky mess out here." BRRRPPP! BRRRRPPPP!

The Blubbaheads started coughing and choking, holding their noses with one hand and fanning the air with the other.

"Whew! That smells like rotten eggs and moldy cheese wrapped in week old fish! Boss, you gotta warn us when you're going to blast that nasty gas!" Faz squawked.

"Oh, zip your greasy lips! This is no time to whine about a little gas." Beads of sweat exploded off Stuffin-Gutt's forehead like popcorn in a microwave oven set on high. He raised his dingy white hanky in the air. "Okay, okay CK, you win. We'll just leave quietly, but please keep that healthy stuff to yourself."

"Not so fast, my junk-food-pushing 'pal'. First, apologize to Danny for baiting him with your fat and greasy garbage. Then promise him you won't ever do it again."

Mr. Stuffin-Gutt rolled his frog eyes to the sky, stroked all three of his chins, and mumbled, "All right, you gotta deal."

CK waved to Danny, "Come on down, Mr. Stuffin-Gutt has something to tell you."

Danny scurried down the stairs and zoomed through the front door. "I can't wait to hear this."

Stuffin-Gutt lowered his head, and his normally strong, booming voice became a quivering whimper. "I...um...I'm sorry for offering you all those fatty sweets, and *I-promise-it-won't-happen-again.*" The battle-weary gut's eyes looked sadder than his worn-out, muddied bedroom slippers. He dragged himself down Danny's driveway grumbling, "Can you believe it, mates? Lost another chunky-flunky to that pain-in-my-gut Cardio Kidd, and his FFF! He pointed to his middle. "This hurts right here."

The cool, calm Faz-n-Greazy tried to ease Stuffin-Gutt's shame and pain. "Don't even sweat it Big Poppa G. There are plennn-tee more Chunky Ds out here just waiting for us to fatten 'em up."

"You're right Greazy. This war has just begun!" Stuffin-Gutt tilted his head upward like he could sniff the scent of his next victim. "I've got a blubbalicious plan for Sweet-Tooth Sarah. C'mon mates, let's get our grub on at McChubby's All-You-Can-Eat Buffet."

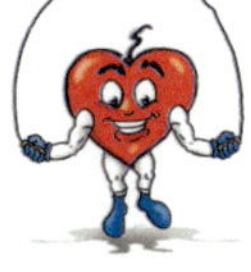

Danny picked up one of the doughnuts from the pile, aimed for the garbage can on the other side of the room, and flicked his wrist like he was shooting a basketball.

"*Sweet* shot!" T-Mac said.

"Thanks! Hey guys, it feels soooooo good to be rid of those tricky Blubbaheads! And now I'm ready to get rid of this jelly belly."

"And you WILL Danny! Right now, though, we need to get rid of ALL this junk food, and clean up this mess before your mom arrives."

Sista Cellie circled her right arm, snapped her long, slender fingers, "Ah Shubeedoowah! *Look at these sky-high stacks of sugary snacks!"* Everyone chuckled and nodded together like bobblehead dolls.

Bonita-B stuffed a monster trash bag so full of candy, chips, cookies, and cheesecake that she could barely drag it out of the house. "Ay T-Mac! I need your strong muscles."

"No problema, mi amiga!" T-Mac replied.

"Man, chasing off the baddies and helping me clean up too! You guys really got my back!"

"We got your back, your arms and legs too—we'll help you strengthen them all! Let's meet tomorrow after school at the Fit-Mobile. To get you fired up for your new fitness journey, we've cooked up one jammin' surprise. And we'll 'wrap' it real tight to keep it fresh for a long time," CK said.

"Oh yeah! I love surprises, especially homemade ones. I'll be there!"

This time the look of firm determination in Danny's eyes told CK that no bullies or Blubbaheads could stop him.

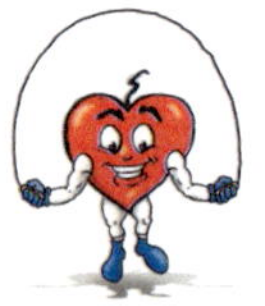

CHAPTER 7: Getting Back in the Game!

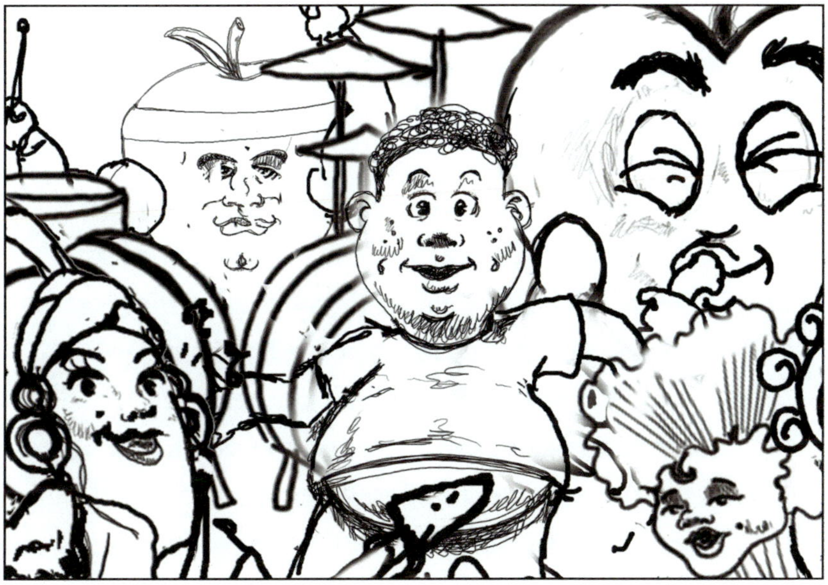

Choice, Choice— It's All About Choice...

Danny swiveled his eyes side-to-side,
from his teacher to the clock.
He'd soon get the biggest surprise of his life
and become the happiest kid on the block!

Danny had just about worn a hole in the seat of his pants with his fidgeting, as he tried to guess what the *jammin' surprise* might be. When the final bell rang, he leaped out of his chair and was already past the school's entrance before the ringing faded. He took off running until his rapid heartbeat forced him to walk. Once his heartbeat slowed, he picked up the pace again. When Danny arrived at the Fit-Mobile, he walked right in.

"Danny, you're here early. And dripping with sweat, are you okay?" CK asked.

"I'm...I'm...great! I...I just need...to catch, catch my...breath. I couldn't...wa...wait to get here! Hey CK, what's up with all the musical instruments?"

"Your jammin' surprise—the "Healthy Choices" rap song!" CK replied. "It's Shoooow Time at the Fit-Mobile!"

We wrote a lil rhyme to help you understand,
the healthy life you want is right in your hand.
So sit back and chill, and pay close a-ttention,
helping you improve your life is our in-tention.
Choice, choice, it's all about choice,
when it comes to your health, you do have a voice.
Eat your fruits and veggies at every meal,
They keep your body healthy, improve how you feel.
Apples, bananas, grapes, and cherries,
melon, kiwi, pears, and STRAW-berries...
Carrots, peas, beans, and tomatoes,
spinach, yams, rice, and baked potatoes.
These are healthy food choices you can make,
there are many more, besides candy and cake.
Sugary foods can give your teeth black holes,
and make it hard to reach your basketball goals
Fat and greasy foods are bad for your heart,
they make you too heavy—you know that's not smart!
If you get the munchies or a snack-attack,

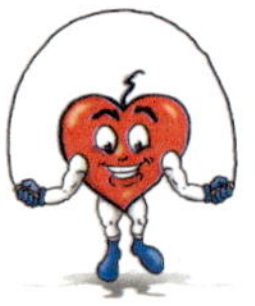

pull a piece of fruit from your school backpack.
When your throat gets dry, to cure your thirst,
say no to pop, drink spring water first.
Push your plate away before your belt gets tight,
take your time Danny boy, enjoy every bite.
Cause it's, choice, choice, it's about choice,
when it comes to your health you do have a voice.
Choice, Choice, it's all about choice,
when it comes to your health you GOTTA have a voice!
Now breakfast is the meal you never wanna skip,
like filling your gas tank before you take a trip.
Now that you're eating healthy everyday,
turn your Xbox off, leave the house and play.
Do what you love, play your number-one sport,
let's shoot, pass, and dribble on the b-ball court.
Stick with the plan, and your day will come,
you'll get picked to play, and have a ton-a-fun.
Cause it's Choice, choice, it's about choice,
When it comes to your health you do have a voice.
Choice, choice, it's all about choice,
When it comes to your health you gotta have a voice!
Don't get up yet, cause we're not through,
we got anotha' rockin' rhyme to rap to you.
After losing weight, you can't get slack,
'cause the Blubba Hill Gang, will surely come back.
They creep late at night, while you're snoozing in bed,
Stuffin-Gutt and his boys will get in your head.
Glazio, Chubba-Chip, Faz-n-Greazy,
wanna tease you, they won't-make-it-easy.
Don't let' em tempt you with a bowl of Chunky Monkey,

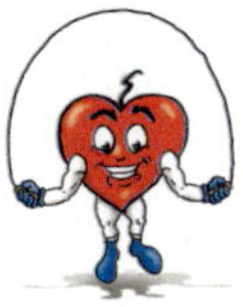

and turn you back into a chubby-food flunky.
The Cardio Kidd and Fat-Fighting Force,
will help you reach your goals and stay on course.
You can do it Danny, you've got-to-be-lieve!
take it day by day, and you will-a-chieve!
Just never make sports more important than school,
'cause failing in the classroom is really not cool
Think for yourself—why follow the crowd?
you wanna be a leader—make your family proud.
If they call you mean names, just smile and wave!
Don't let 'em steal your joy. You've GOT to be brave.
One more point, to please consider,
there are other young people that need to get fitter.
If they come to you and ask for your advice,
share what you've learned, cause it pays to be nice!
We hope this lil rhyme helped you understand,
the healthy life you want, is right in your hand.
Your lesson is over now, things should be clearer,
the only one can stop you is the person in the mirror.
Choice, choice, it's all about choice,
when it comes to your health, you GOTTA have a voice! ©

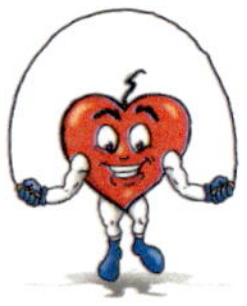

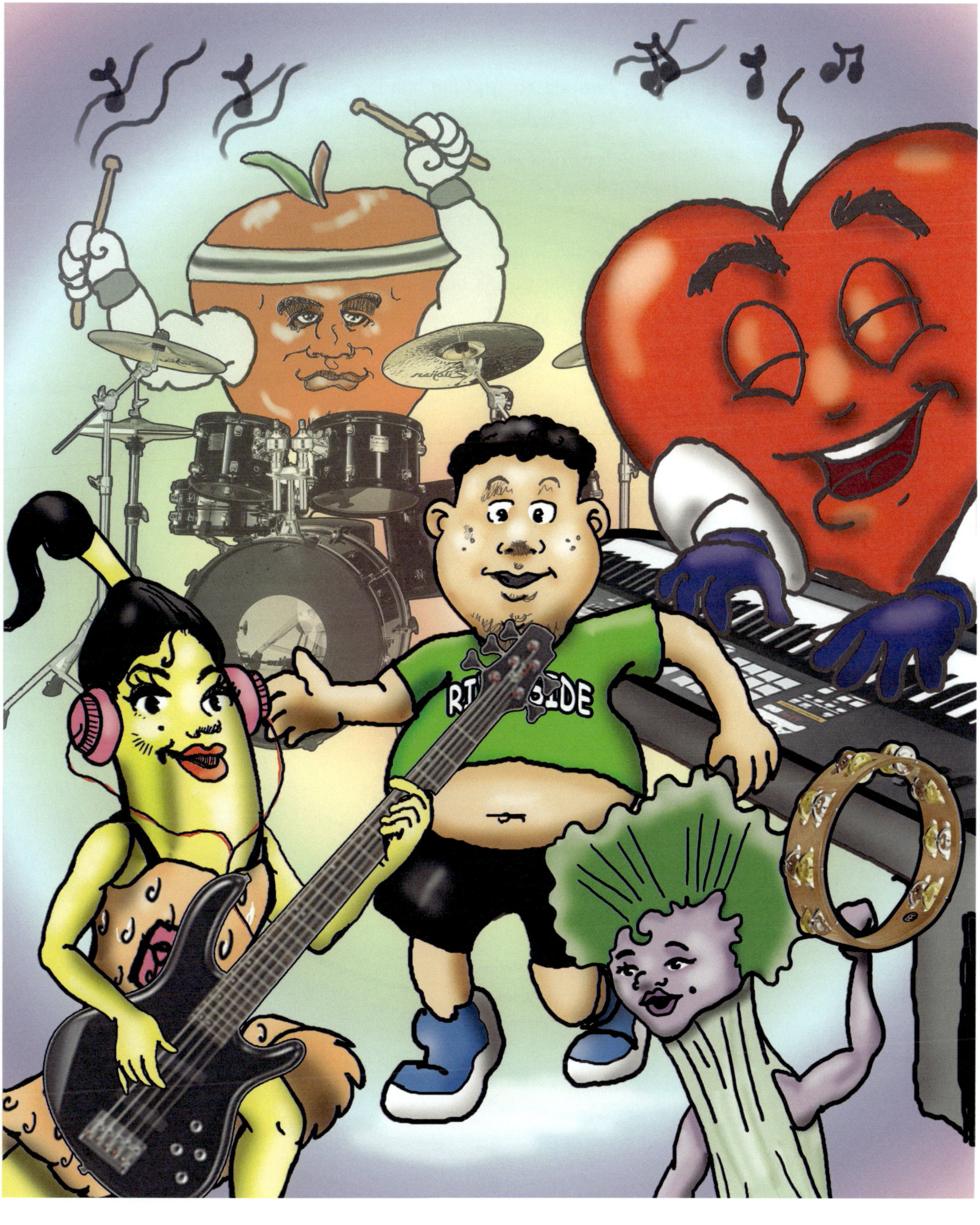

"I love it! I love it!" Danny jumped around the bus like his sneakers had turned into pogo sticks. "Can I get the "Healthy Choices" rap song on a CD?"

"We already thought of that Danny. Bonita-B handed him a small square package. "Here's your special copy signed by CK and the FFF."

"Thanks so much guys!"

As Danny left the bus and headed home, he snapped his fingers, bobbed his head and rapped the song written especially for him. "Choice, choice, it's all about choice, when it comes to your health, you do have a voice!"

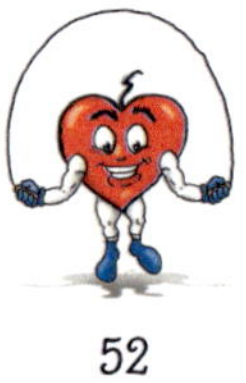

CHAPTER 8:
Getting Back in the Game!

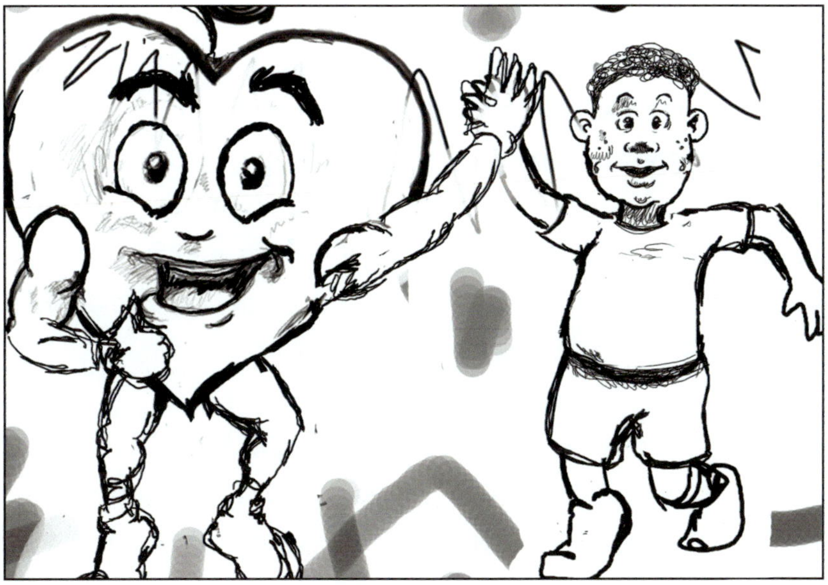

You Gotta Have a Plan, Dan

No high mountain can be climbed alone
or without a great plan.
It takes hard work, belief in yourself,
and a strong helping hand.

"Danny, turn that music down! You'll need a hearing aid before you're fifteen," Mrs. Dixon chided. "Answer the doorbell. Maybe it's your Cardio Kidd friend." She smiled and whispered, "My boy has some colorful imagination. A walking-talking heart with one curly strand of hair."

Danny stumbled over his cat, nearly falling as he scrambled to answer the door. "Come in CK. Mom, meet the Cardio Kidd." When Mrs. Dixon opened her mouth to speak, nothing came out and for once, his chatty mom was tongue-tied.

Danny joked, "Hey Mom, you trying to catch flies?" Danny had to bite his lip to keep from laughing as CK reached out to shake her trembling hand.

"Hello, Mrs. Dixon. I'm CK. It's a pleasure to meet you."

"Uh, it's nice meeting you. Honestly, I thought Danny had dreamed up you and your Fat-Fighting Force from a comic book or cartoon show. But I'm a believer now, and I get why the fitness plan you and Danny put together has him bouncing off the walls. It's been a long time since I've seen my son this happy. And that "Healthy Choices" rap song rocks! Great message! Great beat! Please, have a seat."

"Mom please, you're no Queen Latifah."

"Shush boy. I was rapping before you were born!" Mrs. Dixon teased. "Danny told me how he was bullied yesterday and about that wild water battle with Mr. Stuffin-Gutt, a french fry that glides on grease, a stuttering glazed doughnut and a red-boot-wearing chocolate chip cookie—I would have paid to see that! We laughed all night."

CK chuckled, "Yeah, we cracked up too!"

Then, like a flash of lightening on a sunny afternoon, Mrs. Dixon's mood switched from playful to serious. "I get how important basketball is to Danny, but I worry about him being bullied again, which could mess with his happiness, his health, and then the next thing you know his grades slide. There's no way I'm having that."

CK leaned forward and nodded, "Uh huh, I'm feeling you, Mrs. Dixon."

Danny sat on the edge of his dad's favorite chair, occasionally glancing at the framed photo of him and his dad playing basketball together.

"I love the fitness plan you and Danny put together. No doubt I have to step it up and put the brakes on buying junk food."

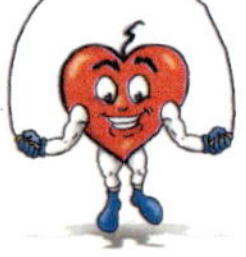

"Yeah, Mom. And you also need to put the brakes on the homemade, hip-sticking cakes and pies."

CK smiled, "I see where Danny gets his quick wit. Look, there's no sugarcoating this, as Danny found out yesterday when he got suckered into a Sugar Bowl Bash by the crafty Blubbaheads. Sticking with this plan won't be easy. But Danny's motivated, and if we work as a team, I know he will improve his fitness level. Then he'll feel and look better, which—in turn—will help him to keep kicking butt in the classroom."

"AND on the basketball court too!" Danny added.

"You're singing my kinda song CK! What a sweetheart!" said Mrs. Dixon, whose deep-dimpled smile mirrored Danny's.

"So Danny, will you be ready to bust a good sweat tomorrow?"

"Do cows moo? I wanna look like Swish and the other players."

"I love your enthusiasm! But understand, people are sort of like fruits and veggies."

"How so?"

"Well, take Sista Cellie, she's long and slender like most celery, right? But she's healthy because she has no brown spots and is crisp not soft or wilted. T-Mac has the opposite shape—he's round and shorter. Why do you think he's healthy?"

"Ummm...because he has no brown spots and is firm?"

"Right! And if he were long and slender like Sista Cellie, he'd be one funny-looking apple, huh?"

"Okay, I get it. I shouldn't try to look like somebody else. I should just live as healthy as possible and be the best me."

"Well said! You learn fast. Eating healthy and doing stuff you enjoy are more important than looking like someone else—make sense?"

"Yes! Hmmm, you're one smart heart CK."

"It was a pleasure meeting you Mrs. Dixon. I'll see you tomorrow Danny."

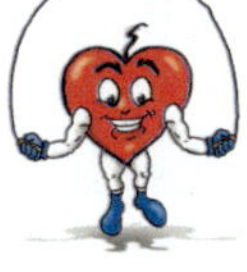

Epilogue:

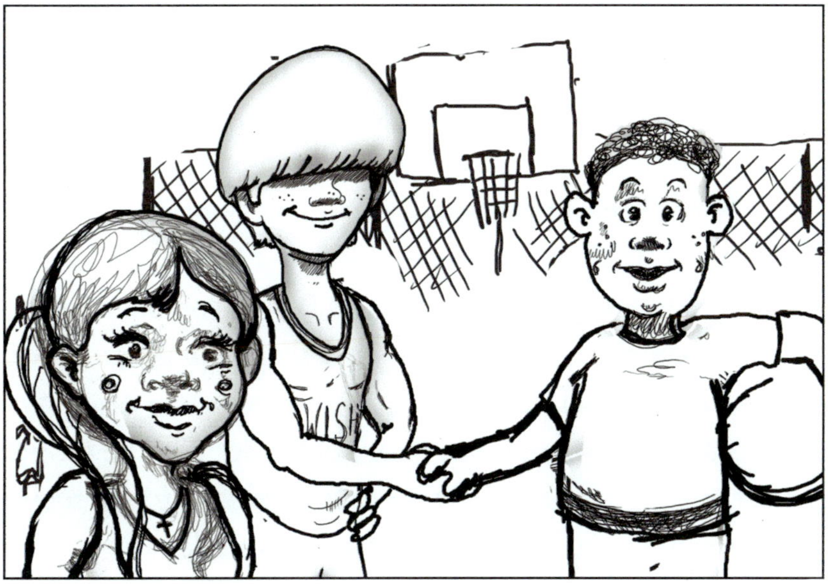

Danny Gets Back in the Game

Danny took the next step,
'cause it was his life to reclaim.
He made the tough choices
and got Back in the Game!

CK and his Fat-Fighting Force met Danny at the park,
they tossed a Frisbee around till it was almost dark.
The first night or two brought on a midnight snack-attack,
but Danny pictured ol' Stuffin-Gutt and said, "Who wants to look like that?"
Dodge ball was a lotta fun, and Danny worked up a big sweat.
Jumping double dutch was tricky, but the most fun yet.
He flew diamond-shaped kites, rode off-road bikes,
and enjoyed Mother Nature's sites on a long, hilly hike.
Did pushups, sit-ups and a bunch of jumpin' jacks,
stretched out real good; ran a mile round the track.
Chased tennis balls and learned how to swim.
They all went roller-skating, and Danny looked more trim.
Mowed grass, raked leaves, and did a few other chores.
Washed the car, did laundry, and helped his mom clean the floors.
Tossing horseshoes was cool but harder than he thought;
the fish were biting good—they returned every one they caught.
Pumping iron with T-Mac made his muscles stronger, and
sprinting with Sista Cellie helped him run faster and longer.
He practiced extra hard on all his basketball skills.
They shot, dribbled, rebounded and worked on passing drills.
Every day they played and learned something new.
Bonita-B showed Danny how to tango and cha-cha too!
Having more fun than ever, he was the happiest kid around,
and then one day his pants kept falling down.
Yes! It was true—his ol' jelly belly had finally shrunk
because he worked so hard and stopped munching on junk.
Running faster, breathing easy, Danny was ready to play ball with the guys.
He was so anxious to return to the park, that night he couldn't close his eyes.

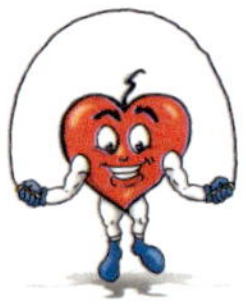

DANNY GETS BACK IN THE GAME

Three months later Danny returned to the park minus his potbelly. Nine players were already shooting around. Danny had been practicing hard on his own everyday, and it showed. As he warmed up alone on the opposite court, he made shots from every angle and distance. His crossover, behind-the-back, and between-the-legs dribbling skills made the other kids stop shooting around and gawk.

"This is the best I've ever felt...can't wait to see the shocked look on Swish's face after he sees me ball," Danny said to himself.

Carmen looked toward Danny and motioned her hand for him to join them. "Hey sharpshooter! We need one more baller, and you got game. Wanna ball?"

Danny's face glowed like a swarm of flashing fireflies. His stomach had that top-of-the-roller-coaster-feeling just before the big drop. He knew this was his big chance to make new friends and once again have a blast playing the sport he was born to play. "Yeah, let's ball!" Danny replied.

A pumped-up Danny missed his first two shots. Then he heard his dad's voice reminding him to breathe deeply and picture the ball going through the hoop. The new slimmer and trimmer Danny used quick spin moves and crafty dribbling to score layups and long-distance shots, and helped his teammates score open shots with pinpoint passing. Like all gifted artists, Danny did things on the court that simply couldn't be taught. All the kids on the sidelines ooohed and ahhhed at his smooth, catlike moves and feathery shooting touch. Across the street CK and the FFF watched the game from the Fit-Mobile. They cheered so loud they started losing their voices. And just as Danny hoped, his team won, and as he often dreamed, all the other players surrounded him like he was a star athlete. But it was Carmen's high-five that meant the most.

"Man, you're the most skilled shooter, dribbler and passer I've ever played with! Are you new to the neighborhood?"

Sweat streamed down Danny's face, his green T-shirt and shorts were soaked. "Sort of," he said with a half-smile.

"I'm Carmen, and this is my bestie Swish. We grew up on these courts."

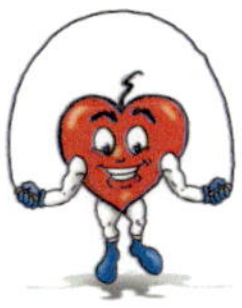

Swish glared at Danny with a *where-have-I-seen-that-face-before-look*. He rubbed his chiseled chin, "Uh huh, that's it! Your face reminds of a pot-bellied wannabe baller that came around a few months ago. Davy or Donny or something. Said he was a top scorer at Riverside. But you can't be that chunky dude," said Swish.

Danny squatted in a Sumo wrestler pose. "Guess what Swish, you're as wrong now as you were the day we met and you grabbed my stomach and called me CHUNKY DAN." He puffed out his cheeks. "Remember me now?" Danny laughed.

Swish's face gushed like he'd just swallowed a red hot chili pepper. And he probably could have stuffed a whole humble pie in his gaping mouth.

For the next few seconds the only sound heard was the faint rustling of a few leaves skipping across the court. Swish looked at Carmen. She nodded her head.

"Uh, hey Danny, I apologize for calling you Chunky Dan and grabbing your stomach. I was wrong. But I really didn't mean to hurt your feelings. I was just teas—"

"Newsflash bro'—WORDS HURT! I felt like walking off a cliff when I left the park that day. But I accept your apology. Like my mom says, we all make mistakes—that's why they put erasers on pencils." Danny turned to Carmen, "Thanks for being nice to me that day. It meant a lot!"

Carmen blushed and replied, "You're welcome Danny!" Then she gave Danny a look he could have poured on a pancake. Danny shook hands with Swish, and then Carmen introduced him to the other players. Suddenly he got a hair-raising, tingly feeling on the back of his neck, like someone was watching him.

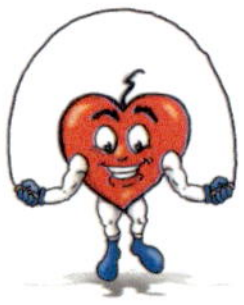

When Danny snapped his head around, he got a surprise sweeter than any sugary glazed doughnut—CK and the FFF were standing just outside the park by the Fit-Mobile watching their happy friend like proud parents. "Hey guys," he said to his new basketball buddies. "I gotta run. I'll see you Saturday."

Danny waved bye and sprinted toward CK, Sista Cellie, Tuffy-McBuffy, and Bonita-B. They all high-fived their special friend with the deep-dimpled smile.

"Yo Danny, you got mad skills!" T-Mac said.

"Thanks! I felt like Iron Man out there, after pumping iron with you."

Bonita-B made a quick cha-cha move; Danny followed with a cha-cha move of his own and spun her around. "The salsa lessons really helped my footwork on the court. Muchos gracias [many thanks], Bonita-B!"

"De nada mi amigo [it's nothing my friend]!" she replied. "We're very proud of you Danny."

He gave Sista Cellie a fist bump. "I'm not gonna lie, I hated running those sprints, but it paid off today. I felt fast and never had to struggle to breathe."

"You worked hard at it. You deserve it! You wanted it! Now, stick with it!" Sista Cellie said.

"I LOVE you guys!"

"We LOVE you too!" they all replied together.

They started walking away from the park when Danny stopped and turned to CK, who had a single tear teetering on the edge of his eyelid, "You were right CK."

CK shrugged, "About what?"

"Binging on junk food. Sitting on my butt all day. Gaining weight...And feeling sorry for myself. It was all about choice—now I'm back in the game!"

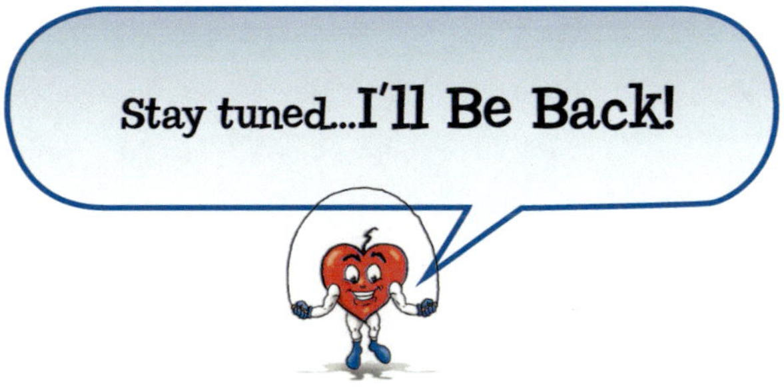

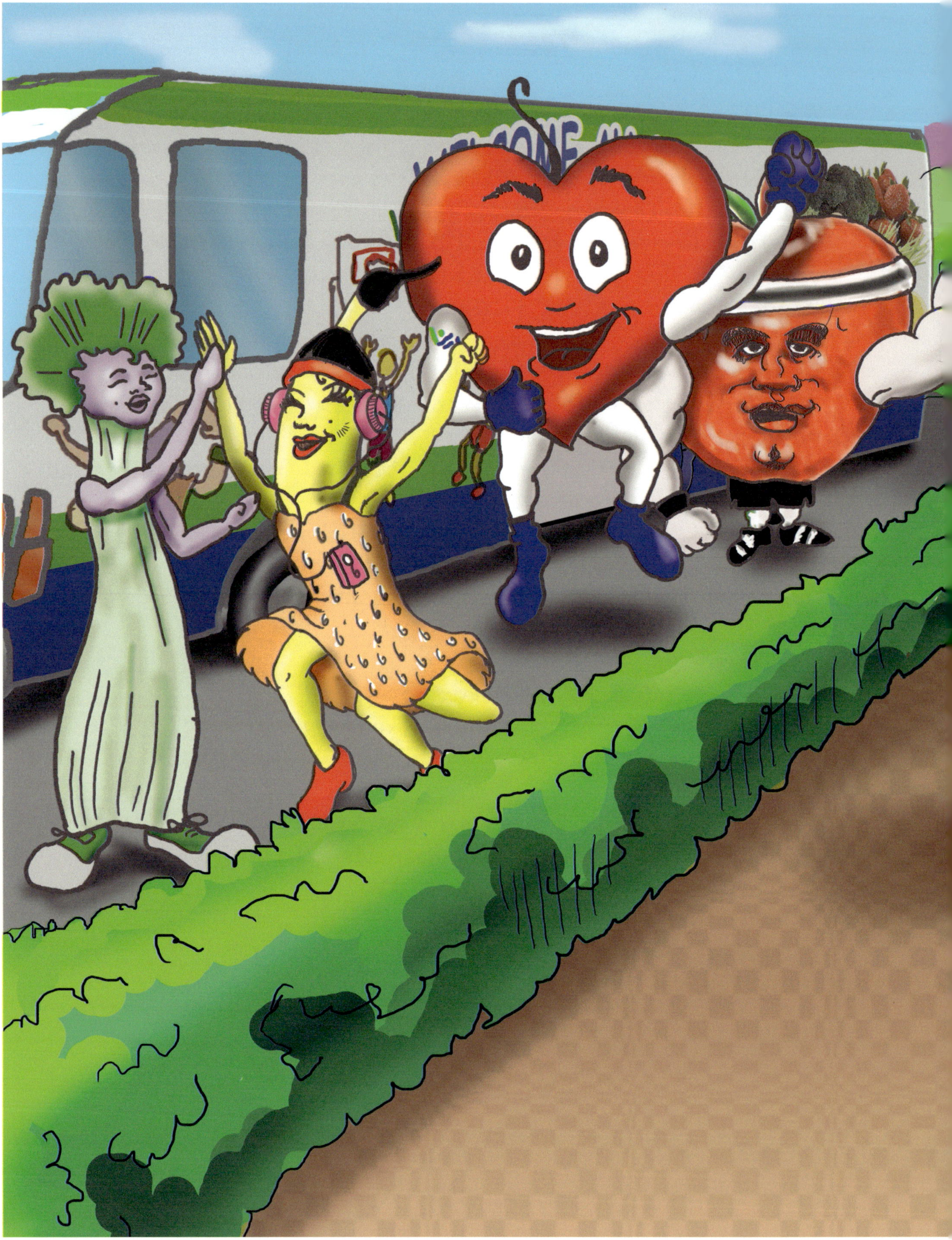

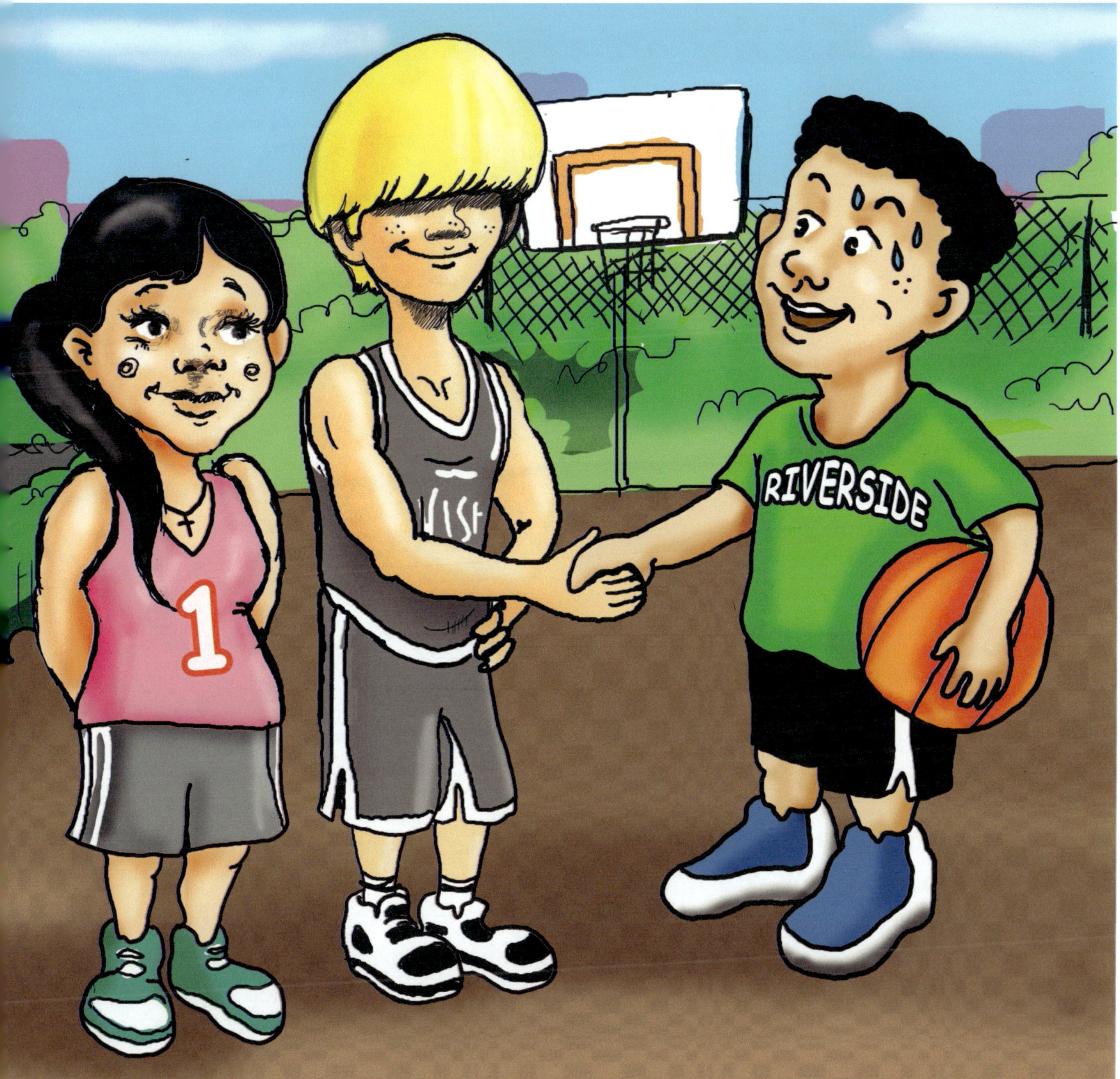

"Uh, hey Danny, I apologize for calling you Chunky Dan and grabbing your stomach. I was wrong. But I really didn't mean to hurt your feelings. I was just teas—"

"Newsflash bro'—WORDS HURT! I felt like walking off a cliff when I left the park that day. But I accept your apology. Like my mom says, we all make mistakes—that's why they put erasers on pencils."

Hello my friend! Thanks for reading *Getting Back in the Game!* But don't stop now—the fun has just begun! To get involved with one or more of IAAC's 2011 Kids Activity Challenges, choose from the below list; you'll have a lotta fun and possibly win a cool prize. For more info go to:

www.cardiokidd.com
and get involved!

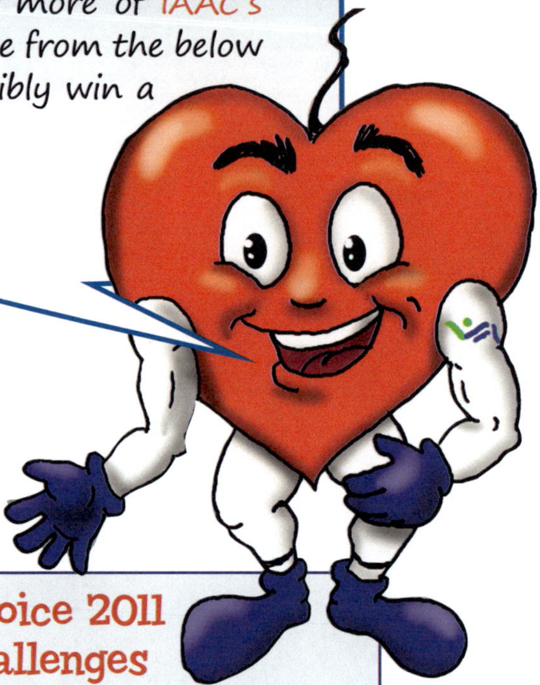

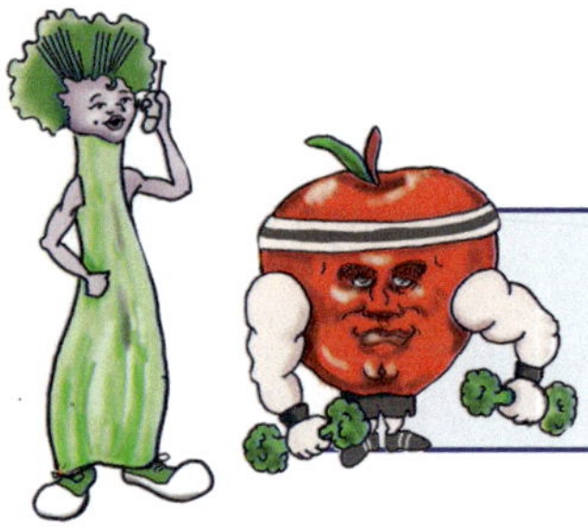

*It's All About Choice 2011 Kids Activity Challenges

- Take our Getting Back in the Game! survey at cardio kidd.com and we will send you one of our cool IAAC Wristbands. We have a unique color band for each of our Fat Fighting Force characters, be the first on your block to collect the entire IAAC set.
- Tell Your Own Story Video Challenge gives you the chance to share why you enjoyed reading Getting Back in the Game! If your video is selected as the top video, win a $100 gift certificate from your choice of Apple, Best Buy, Dick's Sporting Goods, Target or Walmart.
- Create a New Character Contest (for our next book)
- Be the first to start a Cardio Kidd Fan Club
- Can you rap? Sign up for our Healthy Choices Rap Challenge
- If you enjoy writing, sign up for IAAC's Essay Challenge

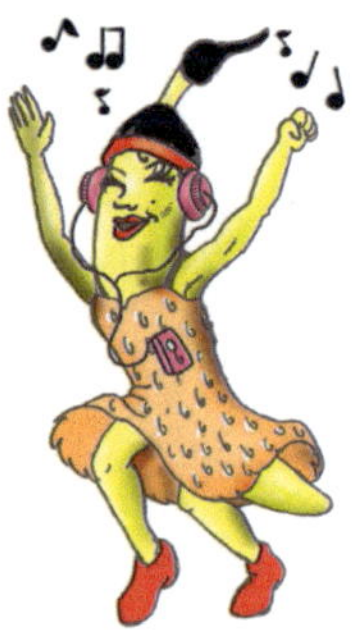

* These Kids Activity Challenges will be offered through the end of 2011. Every year or with each new book, we'll offer new and exciting challenges.

"Yes, Danny became healthier,
and was a real winner on the court.
He also turned bullies into friends,
The true measure of being a good sport!"

APPENDIX I

This section contains discussion points for parents and/or teachers to assist efforts to improve the health of children/students.

Discussion Points:

What could Danny have done differently when he was first bullied at the park?

How did Danny handle the second meeting with Swish? What were the good actions taken by both Danny and Swish? What do you think they both learned from their encounters?

What if Carmen had not been good friends with Swish, would it have been appropriate for her to be just as confrontational with a bully who was a stranger?

Besides not buying sugary snacks, what are some other things Danny's mom could do to help him keep off extra weight?

At what point, if any, should school officials intervene when a student is becoming or is already obese? And what are some things they might do?

If parents or teachers know the name of a child who is bullying other kids, should they attempt to contact and meet with his/her parents? If so, how would you approach this situation?

A possible class project is to have each student bring a food item such as cereal, yogurt, peanut butter, and discuss the nutritional value of each food's individual ingredients. This is a good way to involve kids while promoting an understanding of why reading ingredient labels is essential to maintaining good health.

For more health tips or to participate in our Healthy Choices blog, visit:

www.cardiokidd.com

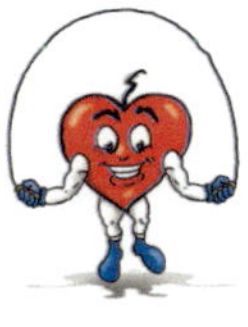

APPENDIX II

IAAC: Healthy Lifestyle Tips

1. Seriously limit soda or other sugar and fat-laden foods and drinks such as ice cream, candy, chips, doughnuts, and cookies and replace them with healthy alternatives such as low-fat yogurt and high-fiber, low-glycemic foods. And lots of water! The fewer sugary and salty foods eaten, the more these foods lose their taste appeal.

2. Increase the variety of fruits and veggies, preferably organic, to daily food choices. This will also boost your immune system. A food journal is one effective way to make sure children eat at least eight to ten servings daily of fruits and veggies.

3. Encourage children to keep their own food journals, as this will help them discover whether or not there's an emotional connection to overeating or junk-food cravings.

4. Make a list of fun games and activities that will keep children active—the other key to shedding extra pounds or keeping them off as they become adults. If they love basketball, sign them up for a pee-wee basketball camp at the YMCA or Boys and Girls Club.

5. If possible don't just drop children off and pick them up later—stay there and cheer them on! They need your encouragement.

6. Make up healthy food cards that can be used for playing learning games or selecting meal choices. It is vital kids understand the importance of different nutrients, and how they help maintain a strong, healthy mind, and body.

7. Keep a daily record of children's work or play activities to ensure they don't play too much and fall behind academically.

8. Make a firm rule that when they ask for food seen on TV that if it's junk food, you won't buy it. You'll eventually get over the NF (Nag Factor) hump.

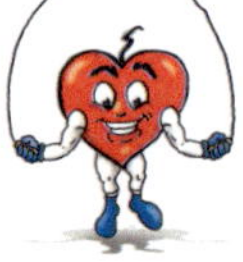

9. Before grocery shopping, have children make a small list of produce items. They'll get physical and mental exercise composing the list, and it's more likely they'll eat the healthy foods from their list.

10. When possible sit together for family meals. Make it an event—a time to share news and tell stories. Eating in front of the TV leads to mindless, unhealthy munching. Put colorful food on the table: green and yellow vegetables, fruits of various colors, and brown (whole-grain) breads. Limit white carbohydrates: rice, pasta, bleached bread, and sugar (desserts).

These common-sense, healthy lifestyle tips are nothing new, yet they are still very effective. Unfortunately, as evidenced by the high childhood obesity rates—worldwide—they are not being followed by a large number of people. The primary goal of *It's All About Choice: Getting Back in the Game!* is to inspire people of all ages to empower themselves (like Danny) to make the challenging choice to eat smarter and become more active. I sincerely hope that goal has been met.

–HDT

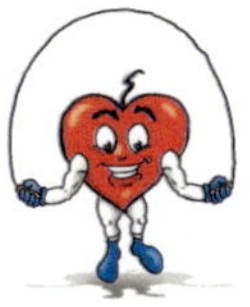

Made in the USA
Monee, IL
05 November 2026

67380475R00050